Patient BILLING

FIFTH EDITION

SUSAN M. SANDERSON

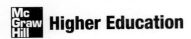

The McGraw-Hill Companies

Higher Education

PATIENT BILLING, FIFTH EDITION

Published by McGraw-Hill, a business unit of The McGraw-Hill Companies, Inc., 1221 Avenue of the Americas, New York, NY 10020. Copyright © 2005, 2002, 1998, 1997, 1995 by The McGraw-Hill Companies. All rights reserved. No part of this publication may be reproduced or distributed in any form or by any means, or stored in a database or retrieval system, without the prior written consent of The McGraw-Hill Companies, Inc., including, but not limited to, in any network or other electronic storage or transmission, or broadcast for distance learning.

Some ancillaries, including electronic and print components, may not be available to customers outside the United States.

 This book is printed on recycled, acid-free paper containing 10% postconsumer waste.

2 3 4 5 6 7 8 9 0 QPD/QPD 0 9 8 7 6

ISBN-13: 978-0-07-301469-2
ISBN-10: 0-07-301469-9

Publisher, Career Education: *David T. Culverwell*
Senior Sponsoring Editor: *Roxan Kinsey*
Managing Developmental Editor: *Jonathan Plant*
Editorial Coordinator: *Connie Kuhl*
Senior Marketing Manager: *James F. Connely*
Senior Project Manager: *Kay J. Brimeyer*
Lead Production Supervisor: *Sandy Ludovissy*
Lead Media Project Manager: *Audrey A. Reiter*
Media Technology Producer: *Janna Martin*
Senior Coordinator of Freelance Design: *Michelle D. Whitaker*
Cover/Interior Designer: *Studio Montage*
(USE) Cover Image: *© Photodisc, Vol. OS 52*
Supplement Producer: *Brenda A. Ernzen*
Compositor: *Carlisle Communications, Ltd.*
Typeface: *11/13.5 Palatino*
Printer: *Quebecor World Dubuque, IA*

Codeveloped by McGraw-Hill Higher Education and Chestnut Hill Enterprises, Inc., Roxbury, CT
chestnuthl@aol.com

The Student Data Disk, illustrations, and exercises in *Patient Billing* are compatible with the NDCMedisoft™ Advanced Patient Accounting software available at the time of publication. Adaptations may be necessary for use with subsequent versions of the software. Text changes will be made in reprints when possible.

All brand or product names are trademarks or registered trademarks of their respective companies.

CPT five-digit codes, nomenclature, and other data are copyright © 2000 American Medical Association. All rights reserved. No fee schedules, basic unit, relative values, or related listings are included in CPT. The AMA assumes no liability for the data contained herein.

CPT codes are based on CPT 2004.

ICD-9-CM codes are based on ICD-9-CM 2004.

All names, situations, and anecdotes are fictitious. They do not represent any person, event, or medical record.

www.mhhe.com

Brief Table of Contents

Contents

Chapter 3:   Managing Data with a Computerized System 39

Chapter 4:   Entering Patient and Case Information 55

Chapter 5:   Processing Transactions 75

Chapter 6:   Processing Claims and Creating Statements 99

Chapter 7:   Producing Reports 115

To the Student

Your Career in Medical Billing

This class introduces you to the concepts and skills you will need for a successful career in medical office billing. Health care continues to be one of the fastest growing industries. As such, there is increasing need for both health care professionals and support staff. One important support function involves the accounting and patient billing aspects of a medical practice. Individuals who have practical experience using patient billing software are well prepared for these challenging tasks. Anyone who aims to get a job in medical billing will find that an understanding of the billing cycle and billing software is often a prerequisite to being hired.

Billing specialists play important roles in the financial well-being of every health care business. Billing for services in health care is more complicated than in other industries. Government and private payers vary in payment for the same services, and healthcare providers deliver services to beneficiaries of several insurance companies at any one time. Medical billing specialists must be familiar with the rules and guidelines of each health care plan in order to submit the proper documentation so that the office receives maximum appropriate reimbursement for services provided. Without an effective billing staff, a medical office would have no cash flow!

To succeed in this field, you will need to possess a variety of abilities and skills. In addition to specialized knowledge about medical billing, you must have computer skills, including database management, spreadsheets, electronic mail, and the Internet. You will also need to possess excellent customer service skills. Even though they are not involved in the actual process of providing medical care, billing specialists come in contact with clients, insurance companies, and patients. For example, incoming calls from patients who have questions regarding a charge are often directed to the billing staff, who must be able to communicate effectively with all types of people.

Medical billing specialist is one of the 10 fastest-growing allied health occupations. This employment growth is the result of the increased medical needs of an aging population and the growing number of health practitioners. Medical billing is a challenging, interesting career, where you are compensated according to your level of skills and how effectively you put them to use. Those with the right combination of skills and abilities may have the opportunity to advance to management positions, such as patient account managers, physician office supervisors, and medical office managers. The more education the individual has, the more employment options and advancement opportunities are available.

About This Book

This text/workbook includes a tutorial and a comprehensive simulation. Once you learn how to operate the NDCMedisoft™ program by completing the tutorial, you can practice those skills by working through the simulation. Both the tutorial and the simulation use a medical office setting, Family Care Center, to provide a realistic environment in which you can learn how to use the software.

NDCMedisoft™ is a popular patient billing and accounting software program. It enables health care practices to maintain their billing data as well as to generate report information. The software handles all the basic tasks that a medical billing assistant needs to effectively perform his/her job. As such, NDCMedisoft™ is an excellent training tool for anyone interested in working as a medical billing assistant. Even if you do not use NDCMedisoft™ on the job, the skills you learn here will be similar to those skills needed to use almost any medical accounting program. You will learn how to perform the following tasks:

- Input patient information
- Enter patient transactions
- Create insurance claims
- Produce patient statements
- Enter payments and adjustments
- Produce reports

Getting Started

Before you jump into the tutorial, review the information provided in this section. Here you will find information that describes the setting and explains your role as a medical billing assistant at the Family Care Center.

Family Care Center

Dr. Katherine Yan, for whom you will work, operates the Family Care Center located in the Stephenson Medical Complex. This medical complex includes suites for 27 doctors, a pharmacy, and a laboratory with X-ray equipment. Like the other medical practices at the Stephenson Medical Complex, the Family Care Center is independently run. Referrals, however, are often made among the physicians in the complex.

Dr. Yan's Office   Dr. Katherine Yan specializes in family practice, which means she is qualified to treat infants, children, and adults. She treats a wide variety of medical conditions such as gynecological problems, cardiac problems, infections, and fractures. Dr. Yan is the first doctor her patients consult for almost any medical problem and for routine physical checkups as well. When patients need more specialized care, such as surgery or obstetrical services for the birth of a baby, Dr. Yan refers her patients to other doctors. Since a variety of specialists have offices in the complex, Dr. Yan is able to send most of her patients to other physicians there. In return, she sees patients who are referred to her by other doctors in the complex.

The office suite that Dr. Yan leases is located just off the landscaped courtyard in the center of the medical complex. Parking is nearby, providing easy access to the office for the physically handicapped patients. The office suite consists of the following rooms:

- A reception area with comfortable furniture and reading materials for adults and children. The office receptionist sits at a workstation in this area. Patients check in here when they arrive and make appointments and pay bills here when they leave. This is where the main office phone is located. The appointment book is kept near the phone so that the receptionist can schedule appointments when patients call the office.

- A spacious office off the reception area with a desk for the medical billing assistant, a computer, a variety of office equipment, and a wall of file drawers. Patient charts, patient financial and medical records, and other records are stored in this area. There is a phone in this area as well, so that the medical billing assistant can handle inquiries from patients and phone calls to patients and insurance companies about their bills and unpaid claims.

- An office for the office manager, next to the medical billing assistant's office.

- An adjacent hallway leading to the following rooms within the office suite: minor surgery room, three examination rooms, small laboratory for routine tests (other tests are performed at the laboratory in the medical complex), office where Dr. Yan speaks with patients, supply room with medical and office supplies, and a rest room.

The office is open Monday, Tuesday, Wednesday, and Friday from 8:00 a.m. to 5:00 p.m. Dr. Yan shares nonoffice-hour calls with six other doctors in the area. She is on call Tuesday evenings and every seventh weekend for emergencies. When Dr. Yan is on call, the members of her staff are also asked to be available in case they are needed.

Members of Dr. Yan's staff include:

- Doris Blackwell—Office Manager. Doris has been with the doctor for the past four years and supervises the business aspects of the practice. She also serves as the accountant for the office, doing payroll, accounts payable, and so on, working closely with a certified public accountant.

- Michelle Walcott—Clinical Assistant. Michelle has worked with Dr. Yan for the past six years. She prepares patients to see the doctor, gives injections, changes dressings, assists in minor surgery, and generally helps the doctor with patient care.

- David Gerardo—Receptionist/Administrative Medical Office Assistant. David handles the front desk and the phones, pulls patients' charts for daily appointments, files the charts, schedules appointments, and orders supplies.

- You—Medical Billing Assistant. Dr. Yan has recently hired you as the new medical billing assistant to replace Bill Larson, who has moved out of the area. Your first responsibility is to learn the NDCMedisoft™ patient billing and accounting software. Although your primary responsibility is for patient records and patient billing, Dr. Yan wants to be sure that you are familiar with the basic accounting system used in the office. The office uses the cash basis for accounting, which means that all revenues are recorded when they are actually received and that expenses are recorded only when they are paid. The patient billing portion of the accounting system has been computerized using NDCMedisoft™ Advanced Patient Accounting.

Your Role   Since one of your major responsibilities is to handle patient accounts in NDCMedisoft™, Dr. Yan has asked that you become familiar with NDCMedisoft™ as soon as possible. You will begin your training by reading materials about how a medical office operates and about how a computerized patient billing system works. The materials will enable you to learn and practice using the various functions of the software before you work with real information.

After you have completed Chapters 1 through 7 of the instructional materials, you will enter patient information for Dr. Yan's office for a four-day period. This will give you an opportunity to work with actual patient information and to try out what you have learned.

How Can I Succeed in This Class?

If you're reading this, you're on the right track.

"You are the same today that you are going to be five years from now except for two things: the people with whom you associate and the books you read."

Charles Jones

Right now, you're probably leafing through this book feeling just a little overwhelmed. You're trying to juggle several other classes (which probably are equally as intimidating), possibly a job, and on top of it all, a life.

It's true—you are what you put into your studies. You have a lot of time and money invested in your education. Don't blow it now by only putting in half of the effort this class requires. Succeeding in this class (and life) requires:

- A commitment—of time and perseverance
- Knowing and motivating yourself
- Getting organized
- Managing your time

This special introduction has been designed specifically to help you learn how to be effective in these areas, as well as offer guidance in:

- Getting the most out of your lecture
- Thinking through—and applying—the material
- Getting the most out of your textbook
- Finding extra help when you need it

A Commitment—of Time and Perseverance

Learning—and mastering—takes time. And patience. Nothing worthwhile comes easily. Be committed to your studies and you will reap the benefits in the long run.

Consider this: your accounting courses are building the foundation for your future—a future in your chosen profession. Sloppy and hurried craftsmanship now will only lead to ruins later.

Side note: A good rule of thumb is to allow 2 hours of study time for every hour you spend in lecture.

Knowing and Motivating Yourself

What type of a learner are you? When are you most productive? Know yourself and your limits and work within them. Know how to motivate yourself to give your all to your studies and achieve your goals. Quite bluntly, you are the one that benefits most from your success. If you lack self-motivation and drive, you are the first person that suffers.

Knowing yourself—There are many types of learners, and no right or wrong way of learning. Which category do you fall into?

- **Visual learner**—You respond best to "seeing" processes and information. Particularly focus on the text's figures and tables.

- **Auditory learner**—You work best by listening to—and possibly tape recording—the lecture and by talking information through with a study partner.

- **Tactile/Kinesthetic Learner**—You learn best by being "hands on." You'll benefit by applying what you've learned during lab time. Think of ways to apply your critical thinking skills in application ways. Perhaps a text website will also help you.

Identify your own personal preferences for learning and seek out the resources that will best help you with your studies. Also, learn by recognizing your weaknesses and try to compensate/work to improve them.

Getting Organized

It's simple, yet it's fundamental. It seems the more organized you are, the easier things come. Take the time before your course begins to look around and analyze your life and your study habits. Get organized now and you'll find you have a little more time—and a lot less stress.

- **Find a calendar system that works for you.** The best kind is one that you can take with you everywhere. To be truly organized, you should integrate all aspects of your life into this one calendar—school, work, leisure. Some people also find it helpful to have an additional monthly calendar posted by their desk for "at a glance" dates and to have a visual of what's to come. If you do this, be sure you are consistently synchronizing both calendars as not to miss anything. *More tips for organizing your calendar can be found in the time management discussion on the next page.*

- **Keep everything for your course or courses in one place**—and at your fingertips. A three-ring binder works well because it allows you to add or organize handouts and notes from class in any order you prefer. Incorporating your own custom tabs helps you flip to exactly what you need at a moment's notice.

- **Find your space.** Find a place that helps you be organized and focused. If it's your desk in your dorm room or in your home, keep it clean. Clutter adds confusion and stress, and wastes time. Or perhaps your "space" is at the library. If that's the case, keep a backpack or bag that's fully stocked with what you might need—your text, binder or notes, pens, highlighters, Post-its, phone numbers of study partners (hint: a good place to keep phone numbers is in your "one place for everything calendar").

A Helpful Hint: add extra "padding" into your deadlines to yourself. If you have an assignment due on Friday, set a goal for yourself to have it done on Wednesday. Then, take time on Thursday to look over your work again, with a fresh eye. Make any corrections or enhancements and have it ready to turn in on Friday.

Managing Your Time

Managing your time is the single most important thing you can do to help yourself. And, it's probably one of the most difficult tasks to successfully master.

You are taking this course because you want to succeed in life. You are preparing for a career. You are expected to work much harder and to learn much more than you ever have before. To be successful you need to invest in your education with a commitment of time.

How Time Slips Away

People tend to let an enormous amount of time slip away from them, mainly in three ways:

1. **Procrastination,** putting off chores simply because we don't feel in the mood to do them right away

2. **Distraction,** getting sidetracked by the endless variety of other things that seem easier or more fun to do, often not realizing how much time they eat up

3. **Underestimating the value of small bits of time,** thinking it's not worth doing any work because we have something else to do or somewhere else to be in 20 minutes or so.

We all lead busy lives. But we all make choices as to how we spend our time. Choose wisely and make the most of every minute you have by implementing these tips.

Know Yourself and When You'll Be Able to Study Most Efficiently

When are you most productive? Are you a late nighter? Or an early bird? Plan to study when you are most alert and can have uninterrupted segments. This could include a quick 5-minute review before class or a one-hour problem solving study session with a friend.

Create a Set Study Time for Yourself Daily

Having a set schedule for yourself helps you commit to studying, and helps you plan instead of cram. Find—and use—a planner that is small enough that you can take with you everywhere. This can be a $2.50 paper calendar or a more expensive electronic version. They all work on the same premise—**organize *all* of your activities in one place.**

Less is more. Schedule study time using shorter, focused blocks with small breaks. Doing this offers two benefits:

1. You will be less fatigued and gain more from your effort, and

2. Studying will seem less overwhelming and you will be less likely to procrastinate.

Plan Time for Leisure, Friends, Exercise, and Sleep

Studying should be your main focus, but you need to balance your time—and your life.

Try to complete tasks ahead of schedule. This will give you a chance to carefully review your work before you hand it in (instead of at 1 a.m. when you are half awake). You'll feel less stressed in the end.

Prioritize!

In your calendar or planner, highlight or number key projects; do them first, and then cross them off when you've completed them. Give yourself a pat on the back for getting them done!

Try to resist distractions by setting and sticking to a designated study time (remember your commitment and perseverance!). Distractions may include friends and surfing the Internet . . .

Multitask When Possible

You may find a lot of extra time you didn't think you had. Review material or organize your term paper in your head while walking to class, doing laundry, or during "mental down time." (Note—mental down time does NOT mean in the middle of lecture.)

Believe it or not, instructors want you to succeed. They put a lot of effort into helping you learn and preparing their lectures. Attending class is one of the simplest, most valuable things you can do to help yourself. But it doesn't end there . . . getting the most out of your lectures means being organized. Here's how:

Prepare Before You Go to Class

Really! You'll be amazed at how much more comprehensible the material will be when you preview the chapter before you go to class. Don't feel overwhelmed by this already. One tip that may help you—plan to arrive to class 5-15 minutes before lecture. Bring your text with you and skim the chapter before lecture begins. This will at the very least give you an overview of what may be discussed.

Be a Good Listener

Most people think they are good listeners, but few really are. Are you? Obvious, but important points to remember:

- You can't listen if you are talking.
- You aren't listening if you are daydreaming.
- Listening and comprehending are two different things. If you don't understand something your instructor is saying, ask a question or jot a note and visit the instructor after hours. Don't feel dumb or intimidated; you probably aren't the only person who "doesn't get it."

Take Good Notes

- Use a standard size notebook, and better yet, a three-ring binder with loose leaf notepaper. The binder will allow you to organize and integrate your notes and handouts, integrate easy-to-reference tabs, etc.
- Use a standard black or blue ink pen to take your initial notes. You can annotate later using a pencil, which can be erased if need be.
- Start a new page with each lecture or note taking session (yes—you can and should also take notes from your textbook).
- Label each page with the date and a heading for each day.
- Focus on main points and try to use an outline format to take notes to capture key ideas and organize sub-points.
- Review and edit your notes shortly after class—at least within 24 hours—to make sure they make sense and that you've recorded core thoughts. You may also want to compare your notes with a study partner later to make sure neither of you have missed anything.

Get a Study Partner

Having a study partner has so many benefits. First, he/she can help you keep your commitment to this class. By having set study dates, you can combine study and social time, and maybe even make it fun! In addition, you now have two sets of eyes and ears and two minds to help digest the information from lecture and from the text. Talk through concepts, compare notes, and quiz each other.

An obvious note: Don't take advantage of your study partner by skipping class or skipping study dates. You obviously won't have a study partner—or a friend—much longer if it's not a mutually beneficial arrangement!

Helpful hint: Take your text to lecture, and keep it open to the topics being discussed. You can take brief notes in your textbook margin or reference textbook pages in your notebook to help you study later.

Getting the Most Out of Your Textbook

McGraw-Hill and the author of this book, Susan, have invested our time, research, and talents to help you succeed as well. Our goal is to make learning—for you—easier.

Here's how:

Patient Billing includes many special features designed to help you master the NDCMedisoft™ billing software. The major features are the following:

The text/workbook is divided into two separate sections—tutorial and simulation. The tutorial lets you learn the basic NDCMedisoft™ software features and the simulation helps you master the program. The tutorial thoroughly describes all of the NDCMedisoft™ options and features that relate to patient billing.

To help you understand these new concepts, the tutorial uses the Family Care Center as a realistic medical office setting in which you perform many of the tasks. Step-by-step instructions guide you through each new activity. Practice exercises begin with simple tasks and progress to more complex activities throughout the tutorial.

The tutorial includes many screen illustrations, source documents, and sample reports to reinforce the concepts introduced in the text/workbook.

Reminders or tips are placed throughout the tutorial. These tips identify shortcuts and list other helpful information for using the NDCMedisoft™ program more effectively.

As you work through a chapter, follow these steps:

- Read the text. Study the figures and screen illustrations that accompany the explanations of various topics.

- As you read, answer the Checkpoint questions that appear throughout the chapter. Write your answers in the text/workbook. Look back at the text if necessary to determine your answer.

- Throughout the tutorial, there are practice exercises that you must complete at the computer. Work through each practice exercise by following the step-by-step instructions. The source documents referred to in the practice exercises are located at the back of the book beginning on page 151.

- Do not skip any practice exercises. You must complete all of the exercises before you begin the simulation.

- If you experience difficulty completing a practice exercise, review the corresponding section in the tutorial and then try the exercise again.

- Complete the chapter review questions after you finish each chapter.

When you have finished Chapters 1 to 7, complete the Patient Billing Simulation by following the instructions beginning on page 133 of the text/workbook. The simulation lets you step into the role of billing assistant for the Family Care Center and apply what you learned in the tutorial to the day-to-day activities of a medical practice. This also provides you with hands-on experience you can take with you into the job market!

To the Instructor

Patient Billing provides your students with the opportunity to learn and perform the duties of a medical billing assistant, using NDCMedisoft™, a computerized patient accounting program. Teaching students how to use a software application such as NDCMedisoft™ can be a challenging endeavor. For that reason, this text/workbook is accompanied by an Instructor's Manual that includes tips, suggestions, and comprehensive information for getting started with the NDCMedisoft™ program.

After you install the software and are ready for your students to begin using the NDCMedisoft™ program, you can rely on the manual for important information that you can use to help your students work through the tutorial. The manual includes chapter-by-chapter teaching suggestions, checkpoint answers, end-of-chapter solutions, and sample printouts corresponding to the practice exercises. Numerous printouts and solutions for the simulation are also provided so that you can check your students' work every step of the way or after they have finished the simulation.

An Instructor's Productivity Center CD-ROM is also included. The CD-ROM contains two tools to enhance the instructional process—an instructor's PowerPoint presentation of Chapters 1-7, and assessment software, an EZ Test Testbank that allows instructors to create, edit, and print customized tests for each chapter.

The CD-ROM also contains a series of end-of-chapter backup files for Chapters 1-7, the Appendix, and the Simulation. These backup files can be used to help teachers evaluate students' work at the end of each chapter. When all exercises for a chapter have been completed, by restoring the backup file for a given chapter, the instructor has easy access to the current state of the exercises. The backup files can also be provided to students who misplace or damage their NDCMedisoft™ working disk during the course of the semester.

McGraw-Hill also offers *Capstone Billing Simulation, 3rd edition.* This text/ workbook is designed to provide students who have completed Patient Billing with a simulated work experience that permits students to integrate acquired billing skills in a realistic manner. In Parts 1 and 2, students learn about the job environment—the physicians in the practice, the work rules, and their role as patient services specialist—and study the practice's Policy and Procedures Manual, which offers a realistic exposure to an actual work setting. In Part 3, On the Job, students complete the work of a billing assistant during a two week on-the-job simulation. Each day's work is clearly presented, and additional NDCMedisoft™ skills are taught in context.

Acknowledgments

For insightful reviews, criticisms, helpful suggestions, and information, we would like to acknowledge the following individuals:

Reviewers of the Fourth Edition

Kay Appenfeldt
Moraine Park Technical College
Fond du Lac, WI

Jo Evelyn Blackwell
Georgia Medical Institute
Atlanta, GA

Pam Burton
Ivy Tech State College
Sellersburg, IN

Shirley J. Eittreim
Northland Pioneer College
Holbrook, AZ

Sheree Hamilton
Tennessee Technology Center
at Shelbyville
Shelbyville, TN

Leslie Heidenreich
NDCMedisoft™ Certified Platinum
Dealer
Pittsburgh, PA

Dorothy Kiel
Lima Technical College
Lima, OH

Loren Korzan
University of Northwestern Ohio
Lima, OH

Cheryl Kowalczyk
Mount Aloysius College
Cresson, PA

Patty Leary
Mecosta-Osceola Career Center
Big Rapids, MI

Marlene Moore
Santa Barbara Business College
Bakersfield, CA

Michelle Sisler
KeySkills Learning, Inc.
Clifton, NJ

William R. Thorn
CHI Institute
Southampton, PA

Reviewers of the Fifth Edition

Roxane Abbott
Sarasota County Technical Institute

Emil Asdurian, M.D.
Plaza College

Marcia Banks
The Chubb Institute, Olympia College

Marion Bucci
Delaware Technical Community
College

Margaret Dutcher
Virginia College at Jackson

Yolanda Beasley Gardner
Bessemer State Technical Institute

Marilyn Graham
Moore Norman Technology Center

Jodee Gratiot, CCA
Rocky Mountain Business Academy

Toni Hartley
Laurel Business Institute

Shawna Benton Harwell
Virginia College

Lisa Hauschild
Ivy Tech State College—Northeast

Cynthia R. Johnson, MLT (ASCP), LMT
Cleveland Institute of Dental Technology

Timothy P. MacDonald
Southern Maine Community College

Mary Jane Montgomery
ETI Technical College

Deborah Mullen
Sanford Brown Institute

Scott A. Norman
Bohecker College

Cindy L. Rosburg
Wisconsin Indianhead Technical Institute (WITC)

Lisa Smith-Proffitt
Hagerstown Community College

Geiselle Thompson
The Learning Curve Plus

Jim Wallace
Maric College—Los Angeles CA Campus

Denise E. Wallen
Academy of Professional Careers

Danny Webb
Golden State College

Stacey F. Wilson, MT/PBT (ASCP), CMA
Cabarrus College of Health Sciences

Cynthia Zumbrun, RHIT
Allegheny College of Maryland

Introduction to Patient Billing

WHAT YOU WILL LEARN

When you finish this chapter, you will be able to:

1. Define the terms introduced in this chapter.
2. Describe the major elements of a manual patient billing system.
3. Explain how patient billing fits into the overall accounting system.
4. Define the financial records a medical billing assistant maintains.
5. Discuss the day-to-day responsibilities of a medical billing assistant.

KEY TERMS

Case Grouping of procedures or transactions, generally organized by the type of treatment or insurance carrier.

Cash payments journal Record of all cash payments, frequently in the form of a checkbook register.

Cash receipts journal Record of all cash received by a business.

CHAMPVA Government health insurance plan for disabled veterans.

CMS-1500 A paper insurance form accepted by government insurance plans in some states and by most private insurers (formerly HCFA-1500).

CPT-4 Listing of codes for medical services or procedures.

Day sheet Daily record of activities, patients treated, fees charged, and payments received.

Diagnosis Physician's determination of what is wrong with the patient, based on an examination.

Encounter form Record of one patient's visit, showing procedures performed, charges, and diagnosis. In a manual system, this document may also be referred to as a fee slip, routing slip, or superbill.

General ledger Record of all the accounts of a business.

Guarantor The person or third party responsible for payment of a patient's medical bills.

ICD-9 Listing of codes for medical diagnoses.

Journal Record of daily transactions listed in chronological order, also known as the book of original entry.

Ledger Group of accounts where debits and credits are posted from the book of original entry.

Medicaid Health insurance offered by the government for low-income people (in California, called Medi-Cal).

Medicare Health insurance made available to elderly and disabled people by the government.

Patient ledger Record of all activity (charges, payments, and adjustments) in an individual patient's account.

Procedure A service performed by a physician or other provider.

Providers Medical staff members, such as doctors and physical therapists, who perform the various services.

TRICARE Government health insurance plan for eligible dependents of military personnel.

Overview of Medical Office Accounting

Like other businesses, a medical office must track the flow of money into and out of the practice. Keeping accurate financial records helps **providers,** the medical personnel who perform the various procedures, make sure that they are properly compensated for the services they perform. Financial data are also important for tax-reporting purposes and are useful in determining whether a practice is profitable.

Medical offices record their financial records in a series of journals and ledgers. A **journal** is a record of the daily transactions listed in chronological order, and a **ledger** shows the activity for each account. The **cash payments journal** lists payments to vendors and employees; and the **cash receipts journal** is used to record any money received.

Patient billing, which involves tracking how much money patients owe and what they have paid, is a key part of a medical office accounting system. The patient billing duties are the primary responsibility of the medical billing assistant. Medical billing assistants maintain records, enter payments, update patient ledgers, prepare patient statements, and process insurance claims. To perform these duties, a billing assistant uses computers and patient billing and accounting software programs.

The **day sheet** (or general journal or daily journal) is a chronological record of all transactions involving patients. From the day sheet, information on the activity in each patient's account can be transferred to the appropriate patient ledger.

Once the billing assistant generates the patient ledgers, the accountant can use this information to update the general ledger. The **general ledger** includes up-to-date balances for all of a medical practice's accounts, and is used to prepare various financial statements, such as an income statement or balance sheet.

Patient Billing

As a medical billing assistant, you will be responsible for all aspects of the patient billing process. On a daily basis, you will most likely maintain various records, enter payments, update patient ledgers, prepare patient statements, and process insurance claims along with other tasks.

This section describes how a billing assistant would perform his or her duties in a manual system without the aid of a computer. The next chapter discusses how a computerized accounting system can be used to make the process more efficient.

Records Kept by the Medical Billing Assistant

A billing assistant must maintain various records that are needed by a practice to operate smoothly. These records include encounter forms, patient cases, day sheets, and patient ledgers.

Encounter Form An **encounter form** (or superbill) is a paper document that lists all services performed for one patient at a single office visit. The form has places for the patient's name, medical services provided that day, diagnosis, amount of each individual charge for that day, total for the visit, and the amount paid. A **diagnosis** is the doctor's determination of what is wrong with the patient, based on an examination.

A sample encounter form is shown in Figure 1-1 on page 4. An encounter form is attached to each patient's chart at the start of the visit. The doctor, lab technician, nurse, or anyone else who performs a procedure for the patient during that visit records the services on the encounter form. A **procedure** is a service performed, such as an office visit with a provider (including examination, evaluation of symptoms, and determination of a course of treatment), an injection, or a laboratory test. At the end of the visit, the assistant at the front desk uses the encounter form to calculate the total charge and to record any payment received. The form then goes to the medical billing assistant, who uses it to update the patient ledger and the day sheet.

Case Many medical offices organize patient records using a case-based system. That is, all patient payments, insurance claim reimbursements, and adjustments are linked to a case. A **case** is a grouping of procedures or transactions generally organized by the type of treatment or insurance carrier. For every new case, a billing assistant must record the pertinent information including the following: case description, guarantor, marital status, employer, provider, insurance carrier, policy number, and diagnosis. The **guarantor** is the person or party responsible for payment of a patient's medical bills.

Day Sheet The day sheet is a list of patients, charges, and services performed each day. In a manual system, a billing assistant must prepare the day sheet from the individual encounter forms and case reports. Day sheets have columns with headings such as "Entry," "Date," "Document," "Description," "Provider," "Code," and "Amount." New charges, payments, and adjustments and the current balance are shown for each patient. A summary of the day's activity appears at the end of the report. (See Figure 1-2 on pages 5–6). Day sheets are used to balance accounts at the end of every month.

Family Care Center
285 Stephenson Boulevard
Stephenson, OH 60089
614-555-0100

7/9/09
DATE

Stanley Feldman
PATIENT NAME

Dr. Katherine Yan
PROVIDER

FELST000
CHART #

OFFICE VISITS - SYMPTOMATIC	
99201	OF--New Patient Minimal
99202	OF--New Patient Low
99203	OF--New Patient Detailed
99204	OF--New Patient Moderate
99205	OF--New Patient High
99211	OF--Established Patient Minimal
99212	OF--Established Patient Low
99213	OF--Established Patient Detailed
99214	OF--Established Patient Moderate
99215	OF--Established Patient High
PREVENTIVE VISITS	
NEW	
99381	Under 1 Year
99382	1 - 4 Years
99383	5 - 11 Years
99384	12 - 17 Years
99385	18 - 39 Years
99386	40 - 64 Years
99387	65 Years & Up
ESTABLISHED	
99391	Under 1 Year
99392	1 - 4 Years
99393	5 - 11 Years
99394	12 - 17 Years
99395	18 - 39 Years
99396	40 - 64 Years
99397	65 Years & Up
PROCEDURES	
12011	Repair of superficial wounds, face
29125	Short arm splint
45378	Colonoscopy--diagnostic
45380	Colonoscopy--biopsy
71010	Chest x-ray, frontal
71020	Chest x-ray, frontal and lateral
73070	Elbow x-ray, AP and lateral

73090	Forearm x-ray, AP and lateral
73100	Wrist x-ray, AP and lateral
73600	Ankle x-ray, AP and lateral
93000	Electrocardiogram--EEG
93015	Treadmill stress test
LABORATORY	
80061	Lipid panel
82270	Hemoccult--stool screening
82465	Cholesterol test
82947	Glucose--quantitative
82951	Glucose tolerance test
83718	HDL cholesterol test
85007	Manual WBC
85025	CBC w/diff.
85651	Erythrocyte sed rate--ESR
86585	Tine test
87040	Strep culture
87430	Strep screen
87086	Urine colony count
87088	Urine culture
INJECTIONS	
90471	Immunization administration
90657	Influenza injection, under 35 months
90658	Influenza injection, older than 3 years
90703	Tetanus immunization
90707	MMR immunization

REFERRING PHYSICIAN   NPI

NOTES

AUTHORIZATION #

DIAGNOSIS
848.9

PAYMENT AMOUNT
$10 copayment, check #2944

Figure 1-1   *Sample Encounter Form*

Patient Day Sheet

Ending 8/29/2011

Entry	Date	Document	POS	Description	Provider	Code	Modifier	Amount
BELHE000		**Herbert Bell**						
95	8/29/2011	0508290000	11		1	04		-15.00
94	8/29/2011	0508290000	11		1	93015		292.50
93	8/29/2011	0508290000	11		1	99212		39.60
		Patient's Charges $332.10		Patient's Receipts -$15.00		Adjustments $0.00		Patient Balance $317.10
BRORA000		**Rachel Brown**						
99	8/29/2011	0508290000	11		1	99211		27.00
100	8/29/2011	0508290000	11		1	83718		31.50
101	8/29/2011	0508290000	11		1	04		-15.00
		Patient's Charges $58.50		Patient's Receipts -$15.00		Adjustments $0.00		Patient Balance $43.50
FELST000		**Stanley Feldman**						
83	8/29/2011	0508290000	11		1	93015		325.00
		Patient's Charges $325.00		Patient's Receipts $0.00		Adjustments $0.00		Patient Balance $325.00
JOHMA000		**Marion Johnson**						
143	8/29/2011	0508290000	11	Blue Cross/Blue Shield	1	BCBPAY		-80.00
75	8/29/2011	0508290000	11		1	93000		70.00
74	8/29/2011	0508290000	11		1	99215		135.00
76	8/29/2011	0508290000	11		1	71010		80.00
		Patient's Charges $285.00		Patient's Receipts -$80.00		Adjustments $0.00		Patient Balance $226.00
MITCA000		**Caroline Mitchell**						
56	8/29/2011	0508290000	11		1	99213		60.00
		Patient's Charges $60.00		Patient's Receipts $0.00		Adjustments $0.00		Patient Balance $60.00
MITHE000		**Herbert Mitchell**		0508290000 11				
105	8/29/2011	0508290000	11	0508290000 11	1	99213		39.00
		Patient's Charges $39.00		Patient's Receipts $0.00		Adjustments $0.00		Patient Balance $39.00
PETAN000		**Ann Peterson**						
107	8/29/2011	0508290000	11		1	03		-10.00
106	8/29/2011	0508290000	11		1	99201		32.00
		Patient's Charges $32.00		Patient's Receipts -$10.00		Adjustments $0.00		Patient Balance $22.00

Figure 1-2 *Sample Patient Day Sheet*

(continued)

Patient Ledger The **patient ledger** lists all the activity for each patient account. To complete this ledger, a billing assistant must manually gather the required information from encounter forms and day sheets. Since some patients do not pay when services are provided, it is very important that the

```
                    Family Care Center
               Patient Day Sheet
                  Ending 8/29/2011

         Total # Patients                    7
         Total # Procedures                  11
         Total Procedure Charges      $1,131.60
         Total Product Charges            $0.00
         Total Inside Lab Charges         $0.00
         Total Outside Lab Charges        $0.00
         Total Billing Charges            $0.00
         Total Tax Charges                $0.00
         Total Charges                $1,131.60

         Total Insurance Payments       -$80.00
         Total Cash Copayments            $0.00
         Total Check Copayments           $0.00
         Total Credit Card Copayments     $0.00
         Total Patient Cash Payments      $0.00
         Total Patient Check Payments   -$40.00
         Total Credit Card Payments       $0.00
         Total Receipts                -$120.00

         Total Credit Adjustments         $0.00
         Total Debit Adjustments          $0.00
         Total Insurance Debit Adjustments $0.00
         Total Insurance Credit Adjustments $0.00
         Total Insurance Withholds        $0.00
         Total Adjustments                $0.00

         Net Effect on Accounts Receivable  $1,011.60


     Practice Totals
         Total # Procedures                 38
         Total Charges                $2,213.70
         Total Payments                -$290.00
         Total Adjustments              -$19.00

         Accounts Receivable          $1,904.70
```

Figure 1-2 *(continued)*

office keep a record of how much each patient owes. The patient ledger report has two purposes:

- It is an internal record that shows the amount each patient owes.

- It serves as the patient statement of account, or bill.

A sample patient ledger is illustrated in Figure 1-3. The patient ledger report includes the patient's name, procedure date and code, provider, charges, payments, adjustments, and account balance.

Family Care Center

Patient Account Ledger

From August 1, 2011 to August 30, 2011

Entry	Date	POS	Description	Procedure	Document	Provider	Amount
BELHE000		**Herbert Bell**		(614)241-6124			
	Last Payment:	-15.00	On: 8/29/2011				
95	8/29/2011			04	0508290000	1	-15.00
94	8/29/2011			93015	0508290000	1	292.50
93	8/29/2011			99212	0508290000	1	39.60
	Patient Totals						317.10
BRORA000		**Rachel Brown**		(614)721-0044			
	Last Payment:	-15.00	On: 8/29/2011				
99	8/29/2011			99211	0508220000	1	27.00
100	8/29/2011			83718	0508220000	1	31.50
101	8/29/2011			04	0508220000	1	-15.00
	Patient Totals						43.50
FELST000		**Stanley Feldman**		(614)555-9295			
	Last Payment:	0.00	On:				
83	8/29/2011			93015	0507280000	1	325.00
	Patient Totals						325.00
JOHMA000		**Marion Johnson**		(614)726-9898			
	Last Payment:	-80.00	On: 8/29/2011				
75	8/29/2011			93000	0507150000	1	70.00
74	8/29/2011			99215	0507150000	1	135.00
76	8/29/2011			71010	0507150000	1	80.00
143	8/29/2011		Blue Cross/Blue Shield	BCBPAY	0507150000	1	-80.00
	Patient Totals						205.00
MITCA000		**Caroline Mitchell**		(614)861-0909			
	Last Payment:	0.00	On:				
56	8/29/2011			99213	0506150000	1	60.00
	Patient Totals						60.00
MITHE000		**Herbert Mitchell**		(614)861-0909			
	Last Payment:	0.00	On:				
105	8/29/2011			99213	0508250000	1	39.00
	Patient Totals						39.00
PETAN000		**Ann Peterson**		(614)555-8989			
	Last Payment:	-10.00	On: 8/29/2011				
107	8/29/2011			03	0507190000	1	-10.00
106	8/29/2011			99201	0507190000	1	32.00
	Patient Totals						22.00

Figure 1-3 *Sample Patient Ledger*

(continued)

Family Care Center
Patient Account Ledger
From August 1, 2011 to August 30, 2011

Entry	Date	POS	Description	Procedure	Document	Provider	Amount
	Ledger Totals						1,011.60
	Accounts Receivable Total						$1,904.70

Figure 1-3 *(continued)*

√CHECKPOINT

1. Which form is also referred to as a superbill?
2. Which ledger is used to track all of the activity for a patient?
3. Which report shows the patients seen, charges recorded, and services performed each day?

Day-to-Day Activities

As a billing assistant, your job is to follow a routine each day to keep the patient accounts up to date. Throughout the month, you must also send out patient statements and process insurance claims.

Recording Information On a daily basis, a billing assistant uses the encounter forms to record case information, identify procedure charges, process patient payments, and make account adjustments. To simplify the billing process, medical offices use a set of standard procedure codes known as **CPT-4** (*Current Procedural Terminology*, Fourth Edition). Procedures that are commonly performed in the practice are usually listed on the encounter form along with the corresponding CPT-4 code. For example, the sample encounter form shown in Figure 1-1 includes several procedure codes such as 82951 (glucose tolerance test) and 85025 (CBC w/differential).These two codes would be marked if the patient received a blood sugar tolerance test and a complete blood count.

As part of the patient case information, you must also record the diagnosis. A set of medical diagnosis codes known as **ICD-9** (*International Classification of Diseases*, Ninth Revision) makes this task much easier. For instance, if a doctor wrote "diabetes mellitus" on a patient's encounter form, you would use the code for diabetes mellitus (250.00) to record the diagnosis.

Entering Payments Every day, as a billing assistant, you will record all payments received from patients and their insurance carriers. You will record these receipts on a day sheet and on the appropriate patient ledgers.

Preparing the Bank Deposit In some medical offices, you may also be responsible for preparing a bank deposit. Each day you will record all of the checks and cash received on a deposit slip, and then take the deposit to the bank. To verify that you recorded the day's receipts correctly, you can compare the bank deposit total with the day sheet total. The totals should match.

Preparing Patient Statements Usually, a billing assistant prepares and mails patient statements once a month. The statements summarize the office visits and charges during the month, itemize payments on the account, and show the unpaid account balance. The statement is the patient's bill for services. In some practices, statements are sent on several days during each month. For example, patients whose last names begin with A to M may be billed on the fifteenth of the month, and patients with last names beginning with N to Z may be billed on the last day of the month. Spreading out the billing means there is less work to be done on one day and that payments from patients will be distributed more evenly throughout the month.

Creating Insurance Claims Very few patients pay all of their medical bills themselves. Most people have some kind of medical insurance to help cover the costs. A small number of patients file their own insurance claims, often attaching a copy of the encounter form to their claim form. In most cases, however, medical offices file insurance claims directly with carriers. It is the medical billing assistant's job to be sure that those claims are created and sent to the insurance carriers. In addition to indicating the CPT-4 codes and charges on the insurance claim, you will enter some basic information about the patient and a code for the diagnosis. If paper forms are used, most government insurance plans and private carriers accept a standard insurance form, the **CMS-1500** (see Figure 1-4 on page 10). When a remittance advice (RA) is received from the insurance carrier, the billing assistant records payments.

Types of Insurance Carriers Table 1-1 on page 11 shows the principal types of insurance carriers that you will deal with.

In addition, you may deal with workers' compensation, a state-regulated type of insurance covering certain on-the-job injuries, or with automobile insurance in the case of an auto accident.

Maintaining Patient Information

When a new patient comes to the office for the first time, he or she fills out a patient information form that asks for the patient's name, address, employer, insurance coverage, marital status, and so on. When a patient moves, changes jobs, changes insurance carriers, or has other new information, that information must be entered on a patient information form as well. As the medical billing assistant, you must make sure that new and updated information is used in preparing insurance forms and statements. It is good practice to ask the patient to update information at every visit.

CARRIER

HEALTH INSURANCE CLAIM FORM

PICA   PICA

1. MEDICARE   MEDICAID   CHAMPUS   CHAMPVA   GROUP   FECA   OTHER   1a. INSURED'S I.D. NUMBER   (FOR PROGRAM IN ITEM 1)
                                                 HEALTH PLAN BLK LUNG
   (Medicare #) (Medicaid #) (Sponsor's SSN) (VA File #) (SSN or ID) (SSN)   (ID)

2. PATIENT'S NAME (Last Name, First Name, Middle Initial)   3. PATIENT'S BIRTH DATE   SEX   4. INSURED'S NAME (Last Name, First Name, Middle Initial)
                                                             MM   DD   YY   M   F

5. PATIENT'S ADDRESS (No., Street)   6. PATIENT RELATIONSHIP TO INSURED   7. INSURED'S ADDRESS (No., Street)
                                      Self   Spouse   Child   Other

CITY   STATE   8. PATIENT STATUS   CITY   STATE
                                       Single   Married   Other

ZIP CODE   TELEPHONE (Include Area Code)   Employed   Full-Time   Part-Time   ZIP CODE   TELEPHONE (INCLUDE AREA CODE)
            (   )   Student   Student   (   )

9. OTHER INSURED'S NAME (Last Name, First Name, Middle Initial)   10. IS PATIENT'S CONDITION RELATED TO: 11. INSURED'S POLICY GROUP OR FECA NUMBER

a. OTHER INSURED'S POLICY OR GROUP NUMBER   a. EMPLOYMENT? (CURRENT OR PREVIOUS)   a. INSURED'S DATE OF BIRTH   SEX
                                             YES   NO   MM   DD   YY   M   F

b. OTHER INSURED'S DATE OF BIRTH   SEX   b. AUTO ACCIDENT?   PLACE (State)   b. EMPLOYER'S NAME OR SCHOOL NAME
   MM   DD   YY   M   F   YES   NO

c. EMPLOYER'S NAME OR SCHOOL NAME   c. OTHER ACCIDENT?   c. INSURANCE PLAN NAME OR PROGRAM NAME
                                     YES   NO

d. INSURANCE PLAN NAME OR PROGRAM NAME   10d. RESERVED FOR LOCAL USE   d. IS THERE ANOTHER HEALTH BENEFIT PLAN?
                                                                         YES   NO   If yes, return to and complete item 9 a-d.

READ BACK OF FORM BEFORE COMPLETING & SIGNING THIS FORM.
12. PATIENT'S OR AUTHORIZED PERSON'S SIGNATURE I authorize the release of any medical or other information necessary to process this claim. I also request payment of government benefits either to myself or to the party who accepts assignment below.

SIGNED _____   DATE _____

13. INSURED'S OR AUTHORIZED PERSON'S SIGNATURE I authorize payment of medical benefits to the undersigned physician or supplier for services described below.

SIGNED _____

14. DATE OF CURRENT: ILLNESS (First symptom) OR   15. IF PATIENT HAS HAD SAME OR SIMILAR ILLNESS.   16. DATES PATIENT UNABLE TO WORK IN CURRENT OCCUPATION
    MM   DD   YY   INJURY (Accident) OR   GIVE FIRST DATE   MM   DD   YY   MM   DD   YY   MM   DD   YY
                    PREGNANCY(LMP)   FROM   TO

17. NAME OF REFERRING PHYSICIAN OR OTHER SOURCE   17a. I.D. NUMBER OF REFERRING PHYSICIAN   18. HOSPITALIZATION DATES RELATED TO CURRENT SERVICES
                                                                                             MM   DD   YY   MM   DD   YY
                                                                                             FROM   TO

19. RESERVED FOR LOCAL USE   20. OUTSIDE LAB? $ CHARGES
                              YES   NO

21. DIAGNOSIS OR NATURE OF ILLNESS OR INJURY. (RELATE ITEMS 1,2,3 OR 4 TO ITEM 24E BY LINE)   22. MEDICAID RESUBMISSION CODE   ORIGINAL REF. NO.

1. _____ . _____   3. _____ . _____

2. _____ . _____   4. _____ . _____   23. PRIOR AUTHORIZATION NUMBER

24. A DATE(S) OF SERVICE From / To			B Place of Service	C Type of Service	D PROCEDURES, SERVICES, OR SUPPLIES (Explain Unusual Circumstances) CPT/HCPCS MODIFIER	E DIAGNOSIS CODE	F $ CHARGES	G DAYS OR UNITS	H EPSDT Family Plan	I EMG	J COB	K RESERVED FOR LOCAL USE
MM DD YY	MM DD YY											
1												
2												
3												
4												
5												
6												

25. FEDERAL TAX I.D. NUMBER   SSN   EIN   26. PATIENT'S ACCOUNT NO.   27. ACCEPT ASSIGNMENT? (For govt. claims, see back)   YES   NO   28. TOTAL CHARGE $ 29. AMOUNT PAID $ 30. BALANCE DUE $

31. SIGNATURE OF PHYSICIAN OR SUPPLIER INCLUDING DEGREES OR CREDENTIALS (I certify that the statements on the reverse apply to this bill and are made a part thereof.)   32. NAME AND ADDRESS OF FACILITY WHERE SERVICES WERE RENDERED (If other than home or office)   33. PHYSICIAN'S, SUPPLIER'S BILLING NAME, ADDRESS, ZIP CODE & PHONE #

SIGNED _____   DATE _____   PIN#   GRP#

(APPROVED BY AMA COUNCIL ON MEDICAL SERVICE 8/88)   **PLEASE PRINT OR TYPE**   APPROVED OMB-0938-0008 FORM CMS-1500 (12/90),   FORM RRB-1500,
APPROVED OMB-1215-0055 FORM OWCP-1500,   APPROVED OMB-0720-0001 (CHAMPUS)

PATIENT AND INSURED INFORMATION

PHYSICIAN OR SUPPLIER INFORMATION

Figure 1-4   *CMS-1500 Claim Form*

Table 1-1 Types of Insurance Carriers

Carrier	Description
Blue Cross/Blue Shield	Non-profit plans with medical, surgical, and hospital benefits. Payments are often made directly to the provider.
Commercial Insurers	Profit-making medical, surgical, and hospitalization insurance plans. Payments are often made directly to the patient.
Medicare	**Medicare** is government health insurance for the elderly. Part A covers hospital services. Part B partially pays for doctor's services. Payments are made to the provider in most cases.
Medicaid (Medi-Cal)	**Medicaid** is government health insurance for low-income people. Payments are made to the provider.
TRICARE and CHAMPVA	Government health insurance for dependents of certain military personnel (**TRICARE**) and dependents of disabled veterans (**CHAMPVA**). Payments are made to the provider.
Health Maintenance Organization (HMO)	A medical center or group of providers that provides medical services to the patient for a fixed yearly fee. Payments are made to the provider.
Preferred Provider Organization (PPO)	Insurer contracts with a group of providers who agree to provide care based on a predetermined list of charges. The provider bills the PPO directly.

✓CHECKPOINT

4. What reference is used to find a procedure code?

5. What reference can be used to find a list of common diagnoses?

6. What type of form is typically used to process insurance claims?

CHAPTER 1 Review

DEFINE THE TERMS

Write a definition for each term: (Obj. 1-1)

1. Day sheet

   _____

2. Encounter form

   _____

3. CPT-4

   _____

4. ICD-9

   _____

5. Patient ledger

   _____

6. TRICARE

   _____

CHECK YOUR UNDERSTANDING

7. List five important financial records that are kept by a medical office that processes transactions using a manual system. (Obj. 1-2)

   _____

   _____

   _____

8. What is the relationship of the various journals in the medical office to the general ledger? (Obj. 1-3)

   _____

   _____

   _____

9. What is the principal responsibility of the medical billing assistant? What are the two main financial records that the medical billing assistant handles when using a manual system? (Obj. 1-4 and 1-5)

_____

_____

_____

10. Similar information is found on a day sheet and a patient ledger. What is the difference between these two forms? (Obj. 1-5)

_____

_____

_____

11. Who in the medical office fills out the encounter form? Who uses the information on the encounter form and for what purposes? (Obj. 1-5)

_____

_____

_____

12. What manual tasks does the medical billing assistant perform on a daily basis? (Obj. 1-5)

_____

_____

_____

13. What tasks does the medical billing assistant perform on a monthly (or other long-term) basis? (Obj. 1-5)

_____

_____

_____

CRITICAL ANALYSIS EXERCISE

14. From a financial point of view, what is the role and importance of patient billing in the medical office? (Obj. 1-4)

_____

_____

_____

_____

_____

Using the Computer for Patient Billing

What You Need to Know

To complete this chapter, you need to know:

- What the major elements of a medical office accounting system are, and how patient billing fits into the system.
- The main responsibilities of a medical billing assistant.
- What financial records the medical billing assistant maintains, and what each record contains.

What You Will Learn

When you finish this chapter, you will be able to:

1. Define the terms used in this chapter.
2. Describe the data files maintained in a medical billing database.
3. Define the options available in a computerized patient accounting system.
4. Compare a manual patient billing system with a computerized system.
5. Start and exit NDCMedisoft™.
6. Make selections from NDCMedisoft™ menus.

Key Terms

Database Collection of information (data) arranged logically so that it can be stored and retrieved.

Data file Subset of data that is part of a larger database.

HIPAA Security Rule Federal legislation that outlines the administrative, technical, and physical safeguards required to prevent unauthorized access to protected health care information.

Knowledge base Searchable collection of updated information about a topic.

Menu bar Listing of menus within a program, from which options are selected.

NDCMedisoft™ Program Date Date used by the NDCMedisoft™ program to process transactions. Unless specifically set, the program uses the current date stored by the computer.

Toolbar A bar located below the menu bar that provides an alternate method of accessing program options. Icons provide rapid access to program options.

Transactions Charges, payments, and adjustments.

Medical Office Databases

In Chapter 1, you learned that the major documents used or produced in a patient billing system are encounter forms, day sheets, patient ledgers, patient statements, insurance forms, and patient information forms. Important information is recorded on each of these documents, and information from one document is often used in the preparation of others.

In a typical medical office using a manual system, basic information about each patient's visit is:

1. Recorded first on an encounter form.

2. Transferred from an encounter form to a day sheet.

3. Posted from an encounter form or day sheet to the patient ledger.

4. Included on the patient statement for the month.

5. Used in preparing an insurance form for the visit.

All information collected and recorded on the various documents in an office can be considered part of a medical office database. A **database** is a collection of information (data) arranged logically so that it can be stored and retrieved.

In a medical office such as the one described in Chapter 1, where all records are kept manually, the database consists of paper records kept in files. When a computerized patient billing system such as NDCMedisoft™ is used, the database is maintained by the computer. Backup copies of data are filed in the office or offsite so that they can be retrieved in the event of computer problems.

A computerized medical billing program such as NDCMedisoft™ stores these major types of data:

- **Provider Data** The provider database has information about the physician(s) as well as the practice, such as its name and address, phone number, and tax and medical identifier numbers.

- **Patient Data** Each patient information form is stored in the patient database. The patient's unique chart number and personal information—name and address, phone number, birth date, Social Security number, gender, marital status, and employer—are examples of information stored in this database.

- **Insurance Carriers** The insurance carrier database contains the names, addresses, and other data about each insurance carrier used by patients, such as the type of plan. Usually, this database also contains information on each carrier's electronic claim submission.

- **Diagnosis Codes** The diagnosis code database contains the ICD-9 (*International Classification of Diseases,* Ninth Revision, *Clinical Modification*) codes that indicate the reason a service is provided. The codes that are most frequently used by the practice are entered in this database.

- **Procedure Codes** The procedure code database contains the data needed to create charges. The CPT (*Current Procedural Terminology*) codes most often used by the practice are selected for this database. Other claim data elements, such as place of service (POS) and the charge for each procedure, are also stored in the procedure code database.

- **Transactions** The transaction database stores information about each patient's visits, diagnoses, and procedures, as well as received and outstanding payments. **Transactions** in the form of charges, payments, and adjustments are also stored in the transaction database.

Within NDCMedisoft™, each database is linked, or related, to each of the others by having at least one fact in common. For example, information entered in the patient database is shared with the transaction database, linking the two. Information is entered only once; NDCMedisoft™ selects the data from each database as needed.

Information stored in a medical office database is used for a variety of purposes. For example, the patient **data file** is used to update patient ledgers, create patient statements, and prepare insurance claims. When you work with a computerized patient billing system, you may not be aware of how much of the database is being used. The computerized system allows you to retrieve data from and add new data to the database automatically as you work.

Options in a Computerized Patient Billing System

A computerized patient billing system allows you to perform many, if not all, of the tasks performed in a manual system. The menus and submenus in the NDCMedisoft™ system provide access to the program features needed to maintain a patient accounting system.

Title Bar

The title bar lists the program name and the practice name.

NDCMedisoft™ Menu Bar

The NDCMedisoft™ main window, shown in Figure 2-1 on page 18, appears after you start the program. The **menu bar** is the main menu that appears horizontally across the top of a program's window. The menu bar lists the

Figure 2-1   *NDCMedisoft™ Main Window with Menu Bar*

names of the menus in NDCMedisoft™: File, Edit, Activities, Lists, Reports, Tools, Window, and Help. Beneath each menu name is a pull-down menu of one or more options. The options shown in the menu bar represent the categories of features available in the NDCMedisoft™ program. As a medical billing assistant, you will most likely not use all of these options; some are used by other staff members. The information shown in Table 2-1 describes most of the options available in the NDCMedisoft™ program and explains which options a medical billing assistant would use.

As presented in Table 2-1, the NDCMedisoft™ program organizes the program options by category. For example, all of the reports are grouped in the Reports menu. To print the Patient Day Sheet report, you would pull down the Reports menu, choose the Day Sheets option, and then choose Patient Day Sheet. Figure 2-2 on page 22 shows the options in the Reports menu.

Toolbar

The **toolbar,** located just below the menu bar, provides icons for quick access to commonly used program functions. All of the options in the Activities application menu can be selected from the toolbar. Also, many of the Lists menu options, the Custom Report List option, and Help options can be selected by clicking on the corresponding button in the toolbar. Each of the toolbar options is identified in Figure 2-3 on page 22.

Table 2-1	NDCMedisoft™ Menu and Options		

Menu	Options	Description	Used in Billing
FILE			
	Open Practice	Allows you to open a database file for a medical practice. This option is useful if you are using NDCMedisoft™ for more than one practice.	Only indirectly to open a practice database.
	New Practice	Creates a new database for a medical practice.	No, usually others will set up a practice.
	Convert Data	Allows you to convert data from earlier versions of NDCMedisoft™.	No.
	Backup Data	Allows you to back up data.	Yes, for making a backup of a medical practice's database.
	Backup Scheduler	Allows you to schedule regular backups.	Yes.
	View Backup Disks	Lets you view data on a backup disk.	Yes.
	Restore Data	Restores data from a backup disk.	Yes.
	Set Program Date	Changes the date used by NDCMedisoft™ to process data.	Yes.
	Practice Information	Allows you to make changes in an existing practice.	No.
	Program Options	Set backup parameters, startup options, and data entry conventions.	No, most program options will already be configured.
	Security Setup	Set up features to ensure the security of the database.	No, will already be configured.
	File Maintenance	Lets you rebuild a medical office database and perform other maintenance options.	Yes, but only if the database files are damaged or need to be purged.
	Exit	Quits the program.	Yes.
EDIT			
	Cut	All of these options provide editing capabilities while you input data. You can use the cut/copy/paste options to make processing data more efficient.	Yes, while entering data into the system.
	Copy		
	Paste		
	Delete		
ACTIVITIES			
	Enter Transactions	Allows you to record charges to patients for office visits and other procedures. You can enter patient copayments.	Yes.
	Claim Management	Provides options to print claim forms or send them electronically.	Yes.
	Statement Management	Allows you to create and print patient statements.	Yes.
	Enter Deposits/Payments	Allows you to record payments and deposits from patients and insurance carriers.	Yes.

(continued)

Table 2-1 NDCMedisoft™ Menu and Options

Menu	Options	Description	Used in Billing
	Quick Ledger	Displays the ledger of the selected patient.	Yes.
	Quick Balance	Displays a summary of a patient's balance.	Yes.
	Billing Charges	Provides option to add billing charges to a patient's account.	If the practice uses billing charges.
	Appointment Book	Can be used to schedule patient appointments, repeating appointments, or other activities for each provider.	No, other staff members are usually responsible for scheduling.
	Eligibility Verification	Allows a patient's insurance eligibility status to be checked online.	Yes.
	Credit Card Management	Allows the processing of patient credit card payments.	If the practice subscribes to the service.
LISTS	Patients/Guarantors and Cases	The options in the Lists menu allow you to update all of the data files or lists stored in a medical office's database. For example, you would use the Patients/Guarantors and Cases option to add new patient information or to update an existing patient's information.	Yes.
	Patient Recall		
	Patient Treatment Plans		
	Procedure/Payment/ Adjustment Codes		
	MultiLink Codes		
	Diagnosis Codes		
	Insurance Carriers		
	Addresses		
	EDI (Electronic Data Interchange) Receivers		
	Referring Providers		
	Providers		
	Billing Codes		
	Contact List		
	Eligibility List		
REPORTS	Day Sheets	Provides access to reports, including patient ledgers, day sheets, and procedure day sheets. You can also create your own custom reports and bills.	Yes.
	Analysis Reports		
	Aging Reports		
	Collection Reports		
	Audit Reports		
	Patient Ledger		
	Patient Statements		
	Electronic Statements		
	Superbills		
	Custom Report List		
	Load Saved Reports		
	Design Custom Reports and Bills		

(continued)

| Table 2-1 | NDCMedisoft™ Menu and Options |

Menu	Options	Description	Used in Billing
TOOLS	Calculator NDCMedisoft™ Terminal View File Add/Copy User Reports Design Custom Patient Data Statement Wizard Customize Menu Bars System Information Modem Check User Information	Provides access to tools such as a calculator, a utility to view the content of a file, and an option to examine information about your computer.	No, except for the calculator if you need to manually calculate a charge.
WINDOW	Close All Windows Minimize All Windows Tile Windows Horizontally Tile Windows Vertically Show Side Bar Clear Windows Positions Clear Custom Grid Settings	Allows you to switch between windows (e.g., Patient List and Diagnosis List) used by the program.	Not directly; these options are not used in billing.
HELP	Table of Contents How to Use Help Getting Started Upgraders from NDCMedisoft™ for DOS NDCMedisoft™ on the Web Online Updates Show Hints Show Shortcut Keys Register Program About NDCMedisoft™	Provides detailed information about each of NDCMedisoft's™ options. Also, includes information needed to register the program and to identify which version of the NDCMedisoft™ program is being used.	Not directly; the options in this menu provide information to help you use the program more efficiently.

✓CHECKPOINT

1. A new patient visits the office and is treated for allergies. Which option from the Lists menu would you use to enter the patient and case information?

2. You need to print a day sheet at the end of a day. Which option would you choose to print this report?

3. A patient recently changed jobs and is now covered by a health insurance company not listed in the medical office's database. Which option would you choose to add the information for this new health insurance company?

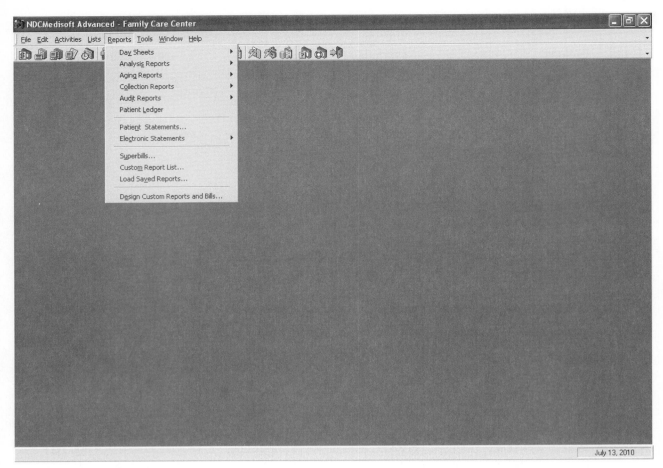

Figure 2-2 *Reports Menu*

Figure 2-3 *NDCMedisoft™ Toolbar*

Getting Started with NDCMedisoft™

Before a medical office begins to create claims using NDCMedisoft™, basic information about the practice and its patients must be entered in the computer. This preliminary work has been done for you. The practice's NDCMedisoft™ databases are stored on the Student Data Disk located inside the back cover of this text. The data are provided in both CD-ROM and floppy disk formats. The medical practice with which you will work is called the Family Care Center.

If you are using the floppy disk, make a copy of it before you begin, using the appropriate set of instructions below. Label the copy "Working Copy." This is the disk that you will use to do the simulations, instead of the original disk. If the copy of your data disk is accidentally damaged or lost or you need to start the simulations over from the beginning, make another copy of the original disk to use as your working copy. Always store the original disk in a safe place.

Making a Copy of the Student Data Disk (floppy disk)

Follow the instructions below to make a copy of the Student Data Disk.

1. Insert the Student Data Disk into the floppy drive (A:).

2. Click on the Start button on the taskbar, and then click on the My Computer icon.

3. Right click on the 3-1/2 Floppy (A:) icon, and then select Copy Disk.

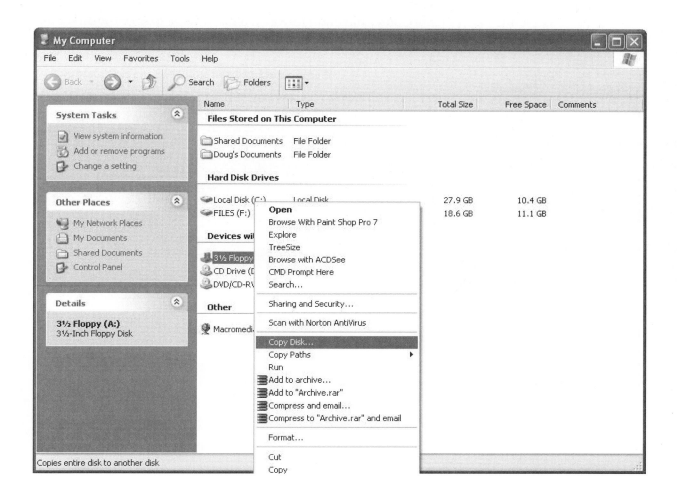

4. In the following window, click on Start to begin the disk copying process.

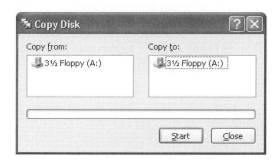

5. When the computer is finished copying data to the new disk, click the Close button and then close the My Computer dialog box.

6. Label the new disk, and store the original disk in a safe place.

Starting NDCMedisoft™

The following instructions take you through the steps of starting the NDCMedisoft™ program the first time the program is used with this text. These steps start the program, create a new directory and data set name for the Family Care Center files, and restore the backup file to the new directory.

1. While holding down the F7 key, click Start, Programs, NDCMedisoft™, NDCMedisoft™ Advanced Patient Accounting to start NDCMedisoft™. When the Find NDCMedisoft™ Database dialog box appears, release the F7 key. (The F7 key bypasses any starting directions that may have been left in the program by a previous user.) This dialog box asks you to enter the NDCMedisoft™ data directory.

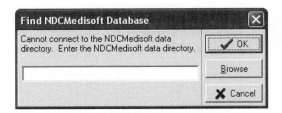

2. Click inside the white data entry box to make it active. Then key **C:\Medidata** in the space provided (where C is the letter that represents the hard drive you will be using). The dialog box should now look like this:

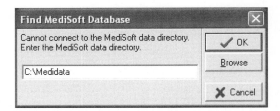

3. Click the OK button. An Information dialog box appears with the following message, "This is not an existing root data directory. Do you want to create a new one?"

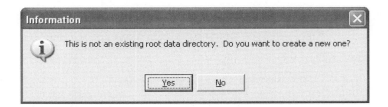

4. Click Yes. *Note:* If a Warning Box appears with information about registering the program, click the Register Later button. The Create Data dialog box is displayed.

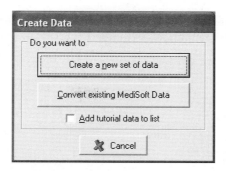

5. Click the Create a New Set of Data button. The Create a New Set of Data dialog box appears. In the upper box, key *Family Care Center.* In the lower box, key *Family.* The dialog box should now look like this:

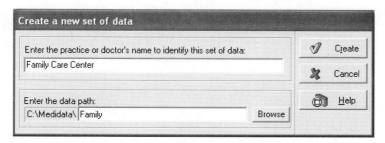

6. Click the Create button. A Confirm dialog box is displayed.

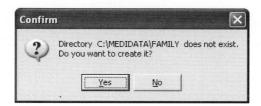

7. Click the Yes button. The Practice Information dialog box appears. In the Practice Name box, key *Family Care Center.* Leave the remaining boxes blank. The dialog box should now look like this:

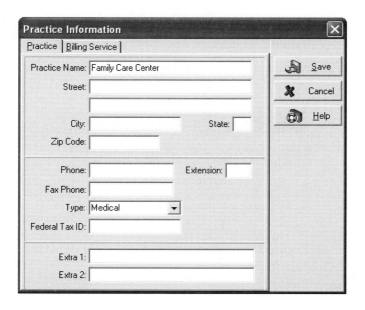

8. Click the Save button. The main window of the NDCMedisoft™ program is displayed. Your screen should look like this:

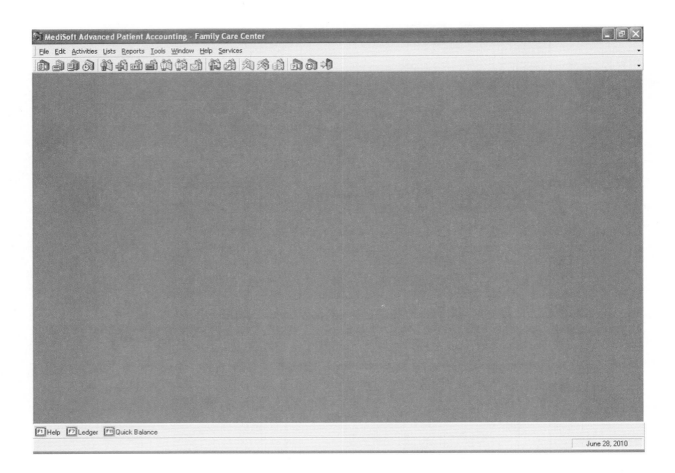

9. Insert the working copy of the Student Data Disk in the floppy drive. (This is usually the A: drive; if your computer uses a different letter to represent the floppy drive, please substitute that letter for *A:* whenever it appears in these instructions.)

10. Open the File menu, and locate the Restore Data option.

11. Click Restore Data. A Warning dialog box is displayed.

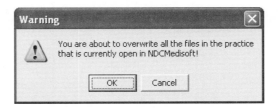

12. Click the OK button. The Restore dialog box is displayed. In the top box, key *A:\PBilling.mbk* if it is not already displayed. The dialog box should now look like this:

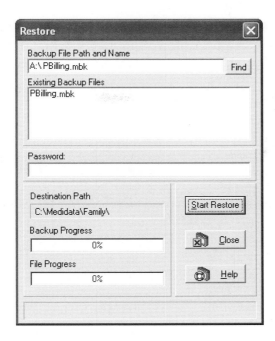

13. Click the Start Restore button. A Confirm dialog box is displayed.

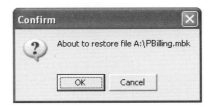

14. Click the OK button. After the program restores the database to the hard drive, an Information dialog box is displayed, indicating that the restore is complete. Click OK.

15. You are returned to the main NDCMedisoft™ window. To open the newly restored data, open the File menu and locate the Open Practice option.

16. Click Open Practice. The Open Practice dialog box is displayed, with the Family Care Center practice name listed.

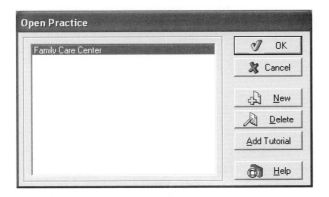

17. To open the Family Care Center database files, click the OK button.

18. The database is now ready for use. (*Hint:* If the main NDCMedisoft™ window does not fill the screen, click the Maximize button to expand it.)

19. To verify that the data has been restored from the Student Data Disk, click Practice Information on the File menu. The Practice Information dialog box should now look like this:

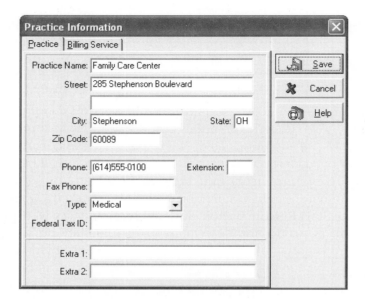

20. Close the Practice Information dialog box.

21. For now, keep the NDCMedisoft™ program open, as it is required in the remaining exercises in the chapter.

Navigating the NDCMedisoft™ Menus

If you are familiar with other Windows applications, you should be comfortable using the NDCMedisoft™ program. Follow the steps in Computer Practice 2-1 to practice choosing options from the application menu.

Computer Practice 2-1: *Using the NDCMedisoft™ Menu Bar*

Follow these steps to choose an option from the NDCMedisoft™ menu.

1. Position the mouse pointer on the Lists menu, and press the left mouse button once to display the menu options.

2. Move the mouse pointer to highlight the Diagnosis Codes option, and then click the mouse button again to select the option.

3. The Diagnosis List window should appear on your screen. Using the options available in this window, you could add, edit, or delete diagnosis codes for the medical practice.

4. Click the Close button shown at the bottom of the Diagnosis List window to close the window.

5. Position the mouse pointer on the Diagnosis Code List button in the toolbar, and then click the mouse button. As you can see, this is another way to open the Diagnosis List window.

6. Close the Diagnosis List window.

7. Click on each of the NDCMedisoft™ menus to view the available options.

Dates

NDCMedisoft™ is a date-sensitive program. If the dates are not accurate when transactions are entered in the program, the data entered will be of little value to the practice. Many times, date-sensitive information is not entered into NDCMedisoft™ on the same day that the event or transaction occurred. For example, Friday afternoon office visits may not be entered into the program until Monday. If the NDC**Medisoft**™ **Program Date** is not changed to Friday's date before entering the data, all the information entered on Monday will be stored as Monday's transactions. For this reason, it is important to know how to change the NDCMedisoft™ Program Date.

For most of the exercises in this book, you will need to change the NDCMedisoft™ Program Date to the date specified at the beginning of the exercise. The following steps are used to change the NDCMedisoft™ Program Date:

1. Click Set Program Date on the File menu, or click the date displayed on the status bar. A pop-up calendar is displayed. (See Figure 2-4.)

2. Click the name of the month that is currently displayed. A pop-up menu appears. Click the desired month on the pop-up menu.

3. Select the desired year by clicking the year that is currently displayed. A pop-up menu appears. Click the desired year on the pop-up menu. For years after 2009, you must select 2009 and then use the right-hand arrow button in the calendar window to advance one month at a time.

4. Select the desired date by clicking on that date in the calendar.

5. The changes to the NDCMedisoft™ Program Date are automatically saved.

Note: The date displayed at the bottom of the calendar labeled "Today" is the Windows System Date—the current date on the computer you are using. Do not click on this date, or the calendar will change to display today's date.

In most NDCMedisoft™ dialog boxes, dates are entered in the MMDD CCYY format. The MMDDCCYY format is a specific way in which dates must be keyed. *MM* stands for the month, *DD* stands for the day, *CC* represents century, and *YY* stands for the year. Each day, month, century, and

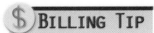

◄		July, 2010				►
Sun	Mon	Tue	Wed	Thu	Fri	Sat
				1	2	3
4	5	6	7	8	9	10
11	12	13	14	15	16	17
18	19	20	21	22	23	24
25	26	27	28	29	30	31

Today: 7/12/2010

Figure 2-4 *Pop-up Calendar*

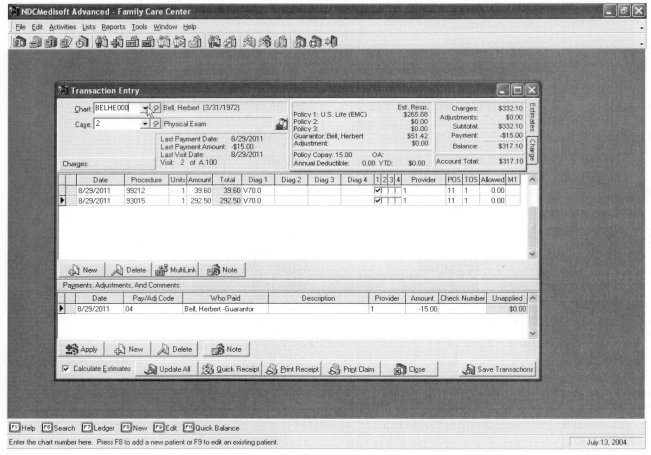

Figure 2-5 **Hints Help Feature**

year entry must contain two digits, and no punctuation can be used. For example, February 1, 2010, would be keyed as "02012010."

Using NDCMedisoft™ Help

NDCMedisoft™ offers users three different types of help.

Hints When the cursor moves over certain fields, text that explains the purpose of the field appears on the status bar at the bottom of the screen (see Figure 2-5).

Built-in Help For more detailed help, NDCMedisoft™ has an extensive help feature built into the program itself, which is accessed through the Help menu.

Online Help The Help menu also provides access to NDCMedisoft™ help available on the NDCMedisoft™ corporate Web site (www.medisoft.com).

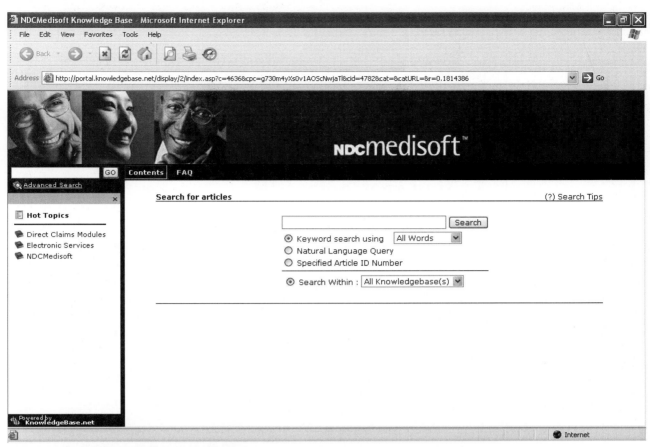

Figure 2-6   *NDCMedisoft™ Online Knowledge Base*

The Web site contains a searchable **knowledge base,** which is a collection
of up-to-date technical information about all NDCMedisoft™ products. (See
Figure 2-6.)

Computer Practice 2-2: *Using NDCMedisoft's™ Built-in Help*

Follow the steps below to use the built-in help feature:

1. Click the Table of Contents option on the Help menu or press
   function key F1. In the left side of the window, NDCMedisoft™
   displays a list of topics for which help is available.

2. Click Diagnosis Entry. Information on entering diagnosis codes is
   displayed on the right.

3. Print the information by clicking the Print button at the top of the
   Help Window. The Print dialog box is displayed.

4. Click the Print button to print.

5. To exit Help, click File on the Help menu bar. Then click Exit.

Computer Practice 2-3: *Using NDCMedisoft's™ Online Help*

Go to NDCMedisoft's™ Web site and explore the knowledgebase.

1. Select NDCMedisoft™ on the Web on the Help menu, and then select Knowledge Base from the submenu.

2. Enter a word or phrase in the Search box, and review the knowledge base entries.

Exiting NDCMedisoft™

When you finish using the NDCMedisoft™ program at the end of each class or lab, you need to back up your data and exit the program. Since you have not made any changes to the database in this chapter, you do not need to make a backup at this time. The topic of backups is covered in the next chapter. After you exit the program, remove the Student Data Disk from the drive and store it in a safe place.

There are three ways to exit the NDCMedisoft™ program:

1. Click Exit on the File menu.

2. Click the Exit Program button on the NDCMedisoft™ toolbar.

3. Click the Close box in the top right corner of the window.

Comparing a Computerized Billing System with a Manual Billing System

As you have learned in this chapter, the NDCMedisoft™ program includes numerous options that can be used by a medical billing assistant to maintain a computerized patient accounting system. A patient accounting program such as NDCMedisoft™ offers many advantages over a manual system. Several advantages of a computerized system are discussed in the following sections.

Access to Information

With a computer database, all the information is located in one place. Pieces of paper and forms are not located in different file cabinets in the office; they are all stored on one computer system.

In addition, computer data can be used by more than one person at a time. If an office has more than one computer, the computers can be linked together in a network, which allows users to share files in the central database. In an office without a computer database, it is difficult for someone to update a document if another person is working on it.

As one security measure, many medical offices assign passwords to individuals who have access to computer files, thereby limiting access to data stored on the computer. Access is granted on an as-needed basis. For example, the individual responsible for scheduling may not be able to access medical records or billing data. On the other hand, the physicians and several others (such as the practice manager) most likely have access to all databases.

As additional security, computer programs keep track of data entry and create an audit trail—a way to trace who has accessed information, and when. When new information is entered or existing information is changed, a log is created to record the time and date of the entry as well as the name of the computer operator. This log is stored and may be reviewed by the practice manager on a regular basis to detect irregularities. In addition, if an error has been made, the program lists the name of the operator and the date the information was entered.

Locating Information

Another advantage of computer databases is the simplicity of conducting a search for information. Instead of having to look in different file cabinets and folders, a search can be conducted by just entering a few keystrokes. In a very short time, the information is retrieved and displayed on the computer screen.

Minimal Storage Space

Computers also eliminate the need for large amounts of physical storage space, since much of the information is stored in the computer, and not on paper.

Productivity

Bringing computers into the medical office has greatly increased productivity, primarily because computers are much more efficient at processing large amounts of data than human beings. Tasks that would take minutes for a human to complete can be done by the computer in a matter of seconds. For example, suppose a medical practice has multiple providers and hundreds of patients. A patient calls to find out the amount owed on an account. With a computerized billing program in place, the medical office assistant might simply key the first few letters of the patient's last name into the computer, causing the patient's account to appear on the screen. The outstanding balance then could be communicated to the patient.

In another example, suppose the wrong diagnosis code has been written on an insurance claim form, and the claim has been rejected by the insurance carrier. To resubmit the claim without the use of a computer might require the entire form to be completed again by hand. However, if the medical office used a computerized billing program, the error could be corrected in seconds and a new claim submitted electronically.

Electronic Claims Processing

An electronic claim is an insurance claim that is sent by a computer over a telephone or cable line using a modem. Today, most insurance claims are transmitted electronically. Electronic claim filing has several advantages. First, filing and processing claims electronically is faster than filling out and processing paper forms and requires fewer staff members. In addition, it costs less to file electronically; the costs of paper forms, envelopes, and postage are much higher than the costs of transmission over telephone lines. Also, chances of error or omission are reduced because information is entered once, not twice. In the case of paper forms, information also has to be entered into the insurance company's computer when the forms arrive by mail.

Fewer Errors

Computers not only make the medical office more efficient; they also reduce the number of errors. Working with a computer system, information is entered once and then used over and over again. Provided the information is entered correctly the first time, it will be correct every time it is used. For example, information such as the patient's address and insurance policy number is entered in the computer once. The computer stores the information, and when the information is needed to create a claim, the computer locates it and uses it to complete the task. The next time a claim needs to be created, the computer goes through the same process, using the same information. Without a computer, someone would have to key all the information on an insurance form each time a claim was being submitted for the patient. Not only does this consume more time, but it introduces the possibility of error every time the information has to be rekeyed.

While computers do increase the efficiency of the medical office and reduce the number of errors, they are not more accurate than the individual entering the data. If human errors occur while entering the information, the data coming out of the computer will be incorrect. Computers are very precise and also very unforgiving. While the human brain knows that *flu* is short for *influenza*, the computer regards them as two distinct conditions. If a computer operator accidentally enters a name as *ORourke* instead of *O'Rourke*, a human might know what is meant; the computer does not. It would probably respond to a request for the ORourke file with the message that "No such patient exists in the database."

Most human errors occur during data entry, such as pressing the wrong key on the keyboard, or because of the lack of computer literacy—not knowing how to use a program to accomplish the tasks. For this reason, proper training in the use of computer programs is essential for medical office personnel.

Claims Processing

From an administrative perspective, the most significant use of the computer in the medical office is to create and process insurance claims. When prepar-

Table 2-2	Manual System versus Computerized System
Manual System	**Computerized System**
Provider fills out an encounter form, and a person at the front desk totals the charge and collects payment.	Same
Medical billing assistant writes the encounter form information on a day sheet.	Medical billing assistant enters the procedure and diagnosis information in the computer.
Medical billing assistant totals columns on a day sheet at the end of a day.	Automatically updated by the program.
Medical billing assistant uses a day sheet at the end of a day to write information on the patient ledgers.	Automatically updated by the program.
Medical billing assistant calculates each patient's new balance.	Automatically calculated by the program.

ing patients' claims, the computer selects information from its databases to create an electronic claim file, which is transmitted electronically.

Fewer Steps to Record Data

One important advantage is that a computerized system eliminates unnecessary steps. For example, NDCMedisoft™ allows you to enter data in one place and then it automatically uses that information in many other areas. Once data has been entered into the system, creating any number of reports is as simple as clicking the mouse.

Table 2-2 identifies the steps to transfer information from the encounter form to prepare a day sheet and a patient ledger. The steps for a manual system are compared with a computerized system. As you can see, many of the steps required in a manual system are performed automatically by a patient accounting program such as NDCMedisoft™.

DEFINE THE TERMS

Write a definition for each term: (Obj. 2-1)

1. Database

   _____

2. Data file

   _____

3. HIPAA Security Rule

   _____

4. Knowledge base

   _____

5. Menu bar

   _____

6. NDCMedisoft™ Program Date

   _____

7. Toolbar

   _____

8. Transactions

   _____

CHECK YOUR UNDERSTANDING

9. List and describe the six major types of data that are part of the NDCMedisoft™ database. (Obj. 2-2)

   _____

   _____

   _____

   _____

   _____

   _____

10. What are the menus listed on the NDCMedisoft™ menu bar? (Obj. 2-3)

_____

_____

_____

_____

_____

_____

11. Which menu includes the option to print a day sheet? (Obj. 2-3)

_____

_____

12. How would you change the NDCMedisoft™ program date to September 8, 2011? (Obj. 2-3)

_____

_____

_____

_____

CRITICAL ANALYSIS EXERCISE

13. Describe the advantages of a computerized billing system over a manual patient accounting system. (Obj. 2-4)

_____

_____

_____

_____

Managing Data with a Computerized System

WHAT YOU NEED TO KNOW

To complete this chapter, you need to know:

- Options available in a computerized system.
- Start-up and exit procedures for NDCMedisoft™.
- Steps to select menu options.

WHAT YOU WILL LEARN

When you finish this chapter, you will be able to:

1. Define the terms used in this chapter.
2. Use the computer keyboard to enter information in NDCMedisoft™.
3. Navigate the NDCMedisoft™ data entry windows.
4. Search for information in NDCMedisoft™.
5. Add a new procedure code to an NDCMedisoft™ database.
6. Create a new chart number for a patient.
7. Back up your data.

KEY TERMS

Backup data A copy of data files at a specific point in time that can be used to restore data to the system.

Chart number A unique number that identifies each patient; in NDCMedisoft™, used on all documents that pertain to that patient.

Removable media device A device that stores data but is not a permanent part of a computer.

Restoring data The process of retrieving data from backup storage devices.

Entering and Editing Data

All data, whether patients' addresses or charges for procedures, are entered into NDCMedisoft™ through the menus on the menu bar or through the buttons on the toolbar. Selecting an option from the menus or toolbar brings up a dialog box. The Tab key is used to move between text boxes within a dialog box. In some dialog boxes, information is entered by keying data into a text box. For example, a patient's name would be keyed directly into a text box. At other times, selections are made from a list of choices already present. For example, when entering the name of the provider a patient is seeing, the name is selected from a drop-down list of providers already in the system.

Editing Data

If you make a mistake entering text in a field, use the Backspace and Delete keys to delete the incorrect text. Then enter the correct information. The Backspace key deletes characters immediately to the left of the cursor. The Delete key deletes highlighted characters, or, if no characters are highlighted, it deletes characters immediately to the right of the cursor.

Saving Data

Information entered into NDCMedisoft™ is saved by clicking the Save button that appears in most dialog boxes (those in which data have been input).

Deleting Data

In some NDCMedisoft™ dialog boxes, there are buttons for the purpose of deleting data. For example, to delete an insurance carrier, the entry for the carrier is clicked in the Insurance Carrier List dialog box. Then, the Delete button is clicked. In most cases, NDCMedisoft™ will ask for a confirmation before deleting the data.

In most dialog boxes, data can also be deleted by highlighting the data and then clicking the right mouse button. A shortcut menu is displayed that contains an option to delete the transaction. Again, NDCMedisoft™ will ask for confirmation before deleting the data. A record of deletions is stored in a database and can be viewed in an audit report.

✓CHECKPOINT

1. How does the Backspace key function when editing data?
2. How does the Delete key function when editing data?
3. How can you delete a transaction from the database?

Computer Practice 3-1: *Entering and Editing Data*

Follow these steps to practice entering information and correcting errors.

1. Start the NDCMedisoft™ program.
2. Set the NDCMedisoft™ Program Date to August 29, 2011.
3. Pull down the Activities menu and select the Enter Transactions option, or click the Transaction Entry button on the toolbar. An empty Transaction Entry window appears as shown in Figure 3-1.

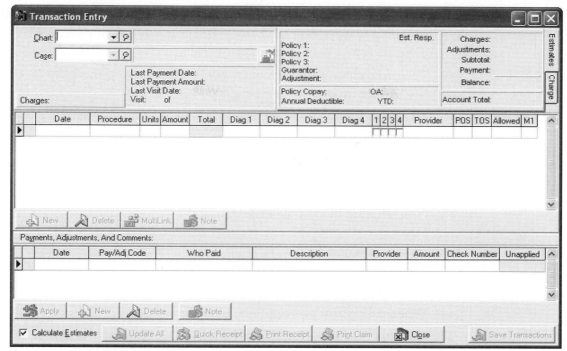

Figure 3-1 *Transaction Entry Window*

4. Key **BE** in the Chart field and press Enter. Information for Herbert Bell is displayed.

5. Make sure that 2 (Physical Exam) is entered in the Case field. If not, enter the case number now.

6. Click the New button in the Payments, Adjustments, and Comments section of the dialog box to enter a new transaction (see Figure 3-2).

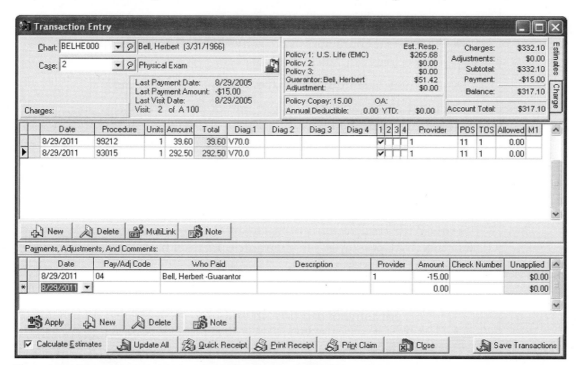

Figure 3-2 *Transaction Entry Window with New Payment Transaction Active*

7. The program automatically enters the date for you.

8. In the Pay/Adj Code field, enter *01* to record a cash payment by a patient. Type the code or select it from the list, and press Enter.

9. The program automatically enters Bell, Herbert in the Who Paid field, since he is listed as the guarantor in this case.

10. Press Tab to move to the Description field, and key Cash Payment.

11. Key *155* in the Amount field, and press Enter. Notice that the program added the decimal point and inserted a minus sign in front of the amount to indicate that it is a payment.

12. Now change the entry in the Amount box to *150.00,* and press Enter.

13. Click the Delete button in the Payments, Adjustments, and Comments section of the dialog box so that you do not record any of the data you just entered.

14. When a Confirm box appears, click Yes.

15. Click the Close button to close the Transaction Entry window.

Patient Chart Numbers

The most important patient information is the chart number (sometimes called an account number). A **chart number** is a unique number that identifies a patient. NDCMedisoft™ requires that you assign an eight-character chart number to each patient.

- A chart number can include any combination of letters (A–Z) and numbers (0–9).

- No special characters such as hyphens, periods, or spaces are allowed (this applies to all data entry fields).

- No two chart numbers in the system can be the same.

Medical practices typically use one of two systems for assigning chart numbers, as described here, but NDCMedisoft™ will automatically assign a chart number using the first system. You can, however, manually assign any chart number you want.

The first system, used by many medical practices and the NDCMedisoft™ program, does not require special coding for the chart number depending on whether a patient is the guarantor (person or party responsible for payment). With this system, bills are mailed to each patient, regardless of whether that person is the guarantor. Here is how a chart number is assigned in this first system:

- The first three characters are the first three letters of a patient's last name.

- The next two characters are the first two letters of a patient's first name.

- The last three characters are 000.

If a new chart number generated by the program matches the first five characters of an existing patient chart number, the program uses 001 for the last three characters, and so on until it finds an available chart number.

The second system assumes that the guarantor (sometimes referred to as the head of household) should receive the bills for all members of a family. Here is how the assignment of a chart number works in this second system:

- The chart number for all members of the same household must have the same first seven characters.

- The guarantor's chart number must end with a zero.

- Chart numbers for other members of a household must end with the digits 1–9.

As with the first system, you may have to make adjustments if there are conflicts with existing codes.

> **$ BILLING TIP**
>
> *Most chart numbers end with three zeros (000), not the letter O. Be sure you enter the chart number correctly.*

✓CHECKPOINT

Using the first method described for assigning chart numbers, identify the chart numbers that the NDCMedisoft™ program would generate for these names.

4. William Jackson

5. Julia Hickson

6. Kim Hwang

Searching in NDCMedisoft™

As you work with the software, you may need to locate information stored in a NDCMedisoft™ database. A computer search allows you to find data that match what you have entered, even if you enter only part of the item. Although you may not need to use this feature very often as you work through this tutorial and simulation, the search feature is especially useful when working with a large database. Some medical practices, for example, have thousands of patients. Using the NDCMedisoft™ search feature, you can search for such things as

- Patient chart numbers

- Insurance carrier codes

- Diagnosis codes

- Procedure codes

- Phone numbers

The search function works differently depending on the context in which you are searching for data, but the same basic guidelines apply. When searching for a patient, insurance company, procedure code, diagnosis code, address, provider, referring provider, or information about a claim,

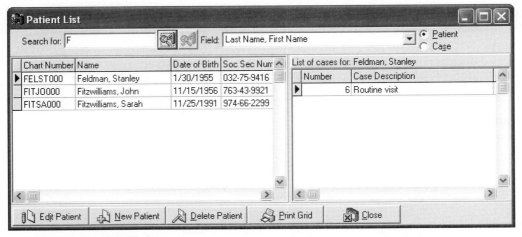

Figure 3-3   *Patient List Window*

the Search For and Field boxes at the top of many windows provide a quick way to find the desired information.

When a character (letter or number) is keyed in the Search For box, the program displays the first instance in the data that matches that character. The options in the Field box control how the list is sorted. To select a different sort option, click the down arrow to the right of the Field box.

Searching for Patients

To begin searching for a patient, you can key the first letter of a patient's last name. As shown in Figure 3-3, keying an *F* in the Search field eliminates all last names that do not begin with the letter *F,* and the selection triangle points to the first chart number that begins with this letter. In our example, the program points to chart number FELST000 (Feldman, Stanley).

As you enter additional characters in the Search field, the program will automatically try to match what you enter with the information stored in its database. Using this technique, you can focus your search even if you don't know a patient's complete name.

The NDCMedisoft™ program lets you search for patients using any of the following criteria: chart number; assigned provider; last name, first name; patient ID #2; last name, first name, middle initial, chart number; Social Security number; and flag.

Searching for Other Data

$ BILLING TIP

Since chart numbers usually begin with the first three letters of a patient's last name, you can use this information to help you quickly locate a patient's chart number.

The NDCMedisoft™ program provides the capability to search for data in almost all of its data entry windows. Whether you need to look up a procedure code that begins with 992 or find a diagnosis code, you can use the search feature to help you locate the information you need. Just enter the information you want to find in a Search field.

Searching for data is not limited to finding information by entering your search criteria in a Search field. The techniques you learned also apply to locating and entering data in a data entry box. As you begin typing characters in a data entry box, the program will display the closest match. Then you can use the arrow keys or your mouse to continue searching in the pop-up list.

Computer Practice 3-2: *Searching for a Patient Chart Number*

Practice searching for a patient chart number following these steps:

1. Select Patients/Guarantors and Cases on the Lists menu or use the appropriate toolbar button.

2. Key the letter *F* in the Search For field to begin your search for Sarah Fitzwilliams' chart number.

3. The program displays a list of patient chart numbers and highlights the first record that begins with the letter *F* (FELST000—Feldman, Stanley).

4. Continue to narrow your search by typing the letter *I* in the field. As you can see, the program highlights the first patient chart number that begins with the letters FI. You could continue to use this method until you find an exact match, or you can select the record once you see it in the list. You could click to highlight Sarah's chart number and then press the desired button at the bottom of the window.

5. Move back to the Search For field and use the Backspace key to erase the letters *FI*. Notice that the full list of patients is displayed.

6. Use the steps you just practiced to search for and select Hal Sampson's chart number.

7. Practice finding other chart numbers.

8. Click the Close button in the Patient List window when you are finished.

Computer Practice 3-3: *Searching for a Procedure Code*

Practice searching for a procedure code following these steps:

1. Pull down the Lists menu and choose the Procedure/Payment/Adjustment Codes option. You can also click the Procedure Codes button on the toolbar. Suppose you want to find the procedure code for a routine exam for an existing (established) patient, but you can only remember that the code begins with 99.

2. Enter **99** in the Search For box as shown in Figure 3-4 on page 46. The program limits the display to codes that begin with the numbers 99.

3. Press Tab three times, and the first item beginning with 99 will be highlighted.

4. Use the arrow keys or click on the scroll bar with the mouse to scan the list of procedure codes. Did you find code 99214?

5. Find the code for an ankle X-ray. The code begins with 73.

6. Click the Close button to close the window.

$ BILLING TIP

Remember to press the Tab or Enter key to move to the next field. If you need to go back to a field, press Shift + Tab.

$ BILLING TIP

You can press the Backspace key in a search box to reset the search criteria so that you can begin again.

$ BILLING TIP

You can also use the Locate (magnifying glass) button in the Transaction Entry window to find a patient or a case. This button is located to the right of the data entry boxes. Selecting this option opens the Patient Search window or Case Search window, where you can search for the specific record you need.

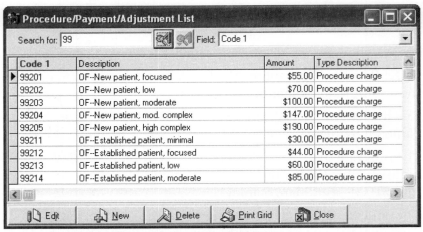

Figure 3-4 *Procedure/Payment/Adjustment List Window*

Adding New Codes

When NDCMedisoft™ is set up in an office, commonly used procedure and diagnosis codes are included in the data file. On occasion, however, you may need to add an additional diagnosis, procedure, or other code to the system.

A variety of codes are routinely used in medical office databases to simplify the data entry process and to standardize the information reported to insurance carriers. When you add a new code, the information you must enter depends on the code itself. For example, when you set up a new procedure code, you must enter the service type and the place where the service was rendered, as well as the charges for the procedure. The standard Type of Service codes and Place of Service codes are shown in Table 3-1 and Table 3-2. Most insurance carriers accept these codes.

Table 3-1	Type of Service Codes			
Code	**Service Type**		**Code**	**Service Type**
1	Medical care		6	Radiation therapy
2	Surgery		7	Anesthesia
3	Consultation		8	Surgical assistance
4	Diagnostic X-ray		9	Other medical
5	Diagnostic lab		0	Blood charges

Table 3-2	Place of Service Codes			
Code	**Place**		**Code**	**Place**
11	Office		22	Outpatient–hospital
12	Home		23	Emergency room–hospital
21	Inpatient–hospital		24	Ambulatory surgical center

Computer Practice 3-4: *Adding a New Procedure Code*

Practice adding a new procedure code by following the steps listed below:

1. Choose Procedure/Payment/Adjustment Codes from the Lists menu, or use the toolbar to select this option.

2. When the Procedure/Payment/Adjustment List window appears, click the New button to add a new procedure code (see Figure 3-5). Notice that there are three tabs: General, Amounts, and Allowed Amounts.

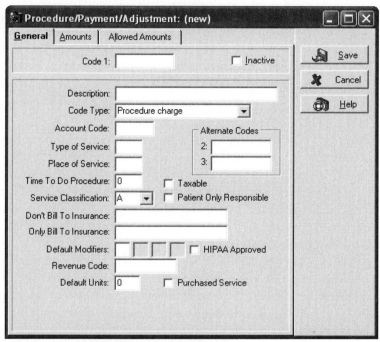

Figure 3-5 *Procedure Code Entry Window*

3. Enter *99402* in the Code 1 field, and then press Tab.

4. Enter *Counseling, limited, 30 minutes* in the Description field.

5. In the Code Type field, choose Procedure Charge if it is not already set.

6. Enter *1* for the type of service. (See Table 3-1.)

7. Enter *11* in the Place of Service field. (See Table 3-2.)

Completing the other fields is optional. The Account Code field, for example, can be used in combination with a medical office's accounting system. The Time To Do Procedure field lets a provider include the number of minutes usually required to perform a procedure.

8. Review the information you entered. If you notice an error, move to the corresponding field to correct the error.

9. Click on the Amounts tab.

10. Enter *50.00* for the charge amount in Box A.

11. Click the Cancel button to close the dialog box without saving your work.

12. Close the Procedure/Payment/Adjustment List window.

Backing Up Data Files

Backup data is the name given to a copy of data files made at a specific point in time that can be used to restore data if the data in the system are accidentally lost or destroyed. In an office environment, you should back up the NDCMedisoft™ data on a regular schedule, usually daily. When data are backed up, they are stored on a removable media device. A **removable media device** is one that stores data, such as a tape or CD-ROM, and is not a permanent part of a computer. Removable media devices may be stored at a location other than the office to protect them from fire or theft. If you use floppy disks, make sure that you have enough formatted disks on hand before you begin the backup process, since you cannot interrupt the program to format a disk.

In an instructional environment, files are also backed up regularly to store each student's work securely and separately. If you are a student working in a computer lab setting, it is important to make a backup copy of your work after each NDCMedisoft™ session. This ensures that you will be able to use your own data during the next session, even if another student uses the computer during the interim or if, for any reason, the data on the hard drive have been changed or corrupted.

In NDCMedisoft™, the Backup Data option on the File menu can be used to make a backup copy of the active database at any time. By default, NDCMedisoft™ also displays a Backup Reminder dialog box when the program is exited. The Backup Reminder dialog box gives you the opportunity to back up your work every time you exit NDCMedisoft™. To perform the backup, the Back Up Data Now button is clicked. To continue to exit the program without making a backup, the Exit Program button is clicked. The following exercise provides practice.

Computer Practice 3-5: *Creating a Backup File When Exiting* NDCMedisoft™

Practice backing up your work on exiting NDCMedisoft™.

1. To exit NDCMedisoft™, click Exit on the File menu or click the Exit button on the toolbar.

2. The Backup Reminder dialog box appears, displaying three options: Back Up Data Now, Exit Program, or Cancel. For the purposes of this text, you will either back up your work to the Student Data Disk in Drive A: or to storage space on a hard drive. The current backup file will overwrite the previous backup file

(A:\PBilling.mbk) on the disk. To begin the backup, make sure your working copy of the Student Data Disk is inserted in Drive A:. Then click Back Up Data Now.

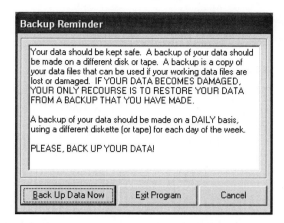

3. The Backup dialog box is displayed. Depending on the last time the dialog box was accessed, the Destination File Path and Name box may already contain the entry A:\PBilling.mbk. If the box is blank, or if it contains something other than this, key *A:\PBilling.mbk* in the Destination File Path and Name box.

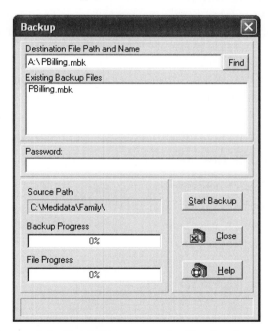

4. NDCMedisoft™ automatically displays the location of the database files to be backed up in the Source Path box in the lower half of the dialog box. Click the Start Backup button.

5. The program backs up the latest database files to the disk in Drive A: and displays an Information dialog box indicating the backup is complete. Click OK to continue.

6. The Backup dialog box disappears, and the NDCMedisoft™ program closes.

Viewing Backup Data Files

Sometimes you need to see what is actually on a backup disk to answer questions such as the following:

- Is this disk the most recent backup?
- Was the backup process performed today?
- Did the backup run correctly?

If the disk you are relying on for backup actually has older data than you want or is defective, it won't do you any good. The View Backup Disks option in the File menu lets you see when the backup file was created, the original data path, how many data files are included in the backup file, and the size of each file.

Restoring the Backup File

The process of retrieving data from backup storage devices is called **restoring data.** Whenever a new NDCMedisoft™ session begins, the following steps can be used to restore the backup file if required. A restore is necessary only if someone else has altered the database files on the hard drive between sessions. If you share a computer in an instructional environment, it is recommended you perform a restore before each new session to be sure you are working with your own data.

To restore A:\PBilling.mbk to C:\Medidata\Family:

1. Start NDCMedisoft™.
2. Check the program's title bar at the top of the screen to make sure the Family Care Center data set is the active data set. (If it is not, use the Open Practice option on the File menu to select it.)
3. Insert your working copy of the Student Data Disk in Drive A:.
4. Open the File menu and click Restore Data.
5. When the Warning box appears, click OK.
6. The Restore dialog box appears. In the Backup File Path and Name box at the top of the dialog box, if the following file name is not already displayed, key *A:\PBilling.mbk.*

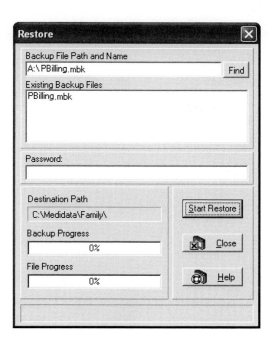

7. The Destination Path at the bottom of the box should already be C:\Medidata\Family. Do not change this.

8. Click the Start Restore button.

9. When the Confirm box appears, click OK.

10. After the files are restored, an Information dialog box appears, indicating that the restore is complete. Click OK to continue.

11. The Restore dialog box disappears. The database has been restored.

Chapter 3 Review

Define the Terms

Write a definition for each term: (Obj. 3-1)

1. Backup data

   _____

2. Chart number

   _____

3. Removable media device

   _____

4. Restoring data

   _____

Check Your Understanding

5. When you enter and edit text, what is the difference between the Backspace key and the Delete key? (Obj. 3-2)

   _____

   _____

6. What chart numbers would you create for these patients—John Jackson, Wilma Smith, and David Wong—when it is not important to identify the guarantor or head of household? (Obj. 3-6)

   _____

   _____

   _____

7. What capabilities does NDCMedisoft™ provide to search for a patient name or other information stored in a database? (Obj. 3-4)

   _____

   _____

   _____

8. Why are codes used in a medical billing program such as NDCMedisoft™? (Obj. 3-5)

_____

_____

9. Explain the steps necessary to add a new procedure code. (Obj. 3-5)

_____

_____

_____

_____

10. What options are available in the NDCMedisoft™ program to facilitate the backup process in a medical office? (Obj. 3-7)

_____

_____

_____

CRITICAL ANALYSIS EXERCISE

11. You are working in an office entering data from Tuesday when a power failure occurs. When power is restored, you find that much of the data in the NDCMedisoft™ system has errors caused by the failure. What should you do? (Obj. 3-7)

_____

_____

_____

_____

Entering Patient and Case Information

WHAT YOU NEED TO KNOW

To complete this chapter, you need to know how to:

- Navigate the NDCMedisoft™ software.
- Search for information in an NDCMedisoft™ database.

WHAT YOU WILL LEARN

When you finish this chapter, you will be able to:

1. Define the terms used in this chapter.
2. Explain the information requirements for a new patient record.
3. Add a new patient account.
4. Describe the information needed for a new patient case record.
5. Enter a new patient case record.
6. Revise patient information.

KEY TERMS

Capitated plan Type of insurance that pays providers a fixed amount for each patient regardless of the actual medical services rendered.

Case billing code A code used to group or organize patients for billing purposes, such as *M* for Medicare or *C* for cash patient.

Copayment Standard fee for medical services rendered, set up by an insurance carrier, that the patient pays to the provider at the time of service.

EPSDT Well-baby program sponsored by Medicaid.

Established patient A patient who has received medical care from the provider in the last three years.

New patient A patient who has never visited the medical office or has not received professional care from the provider in the last three years.

Patient billing code A code that indicates the schedule of fees that apply to the patient.

Patient information form A form completed by a patient that includes personal information such as name, address, employer, insurance company, and any known allergies.

Signature on file Field used to indicate whether a patient's signature is on file.

Type The field used to identify an individual or another party as a patient or a guarantor.

How Patient Information Is Organized

As you already learned, the NDCMedisoft™ program requires that you maintain an up-to-date patient database so that the software can process the billing information efficiently. To keep the patient database current, you will need to add information for new patients and update existing patient records. For medical billing purposes, a **new patient** is a patient who has never visited the office or a person who has not seen his or her provider in the past three years. An **established patient** is someone who has received medical care in the office during the past three years.

When a new patient visits a medical office, he or she must fill out a patient information form similar to the one shown in Figure 4-1. The **patient information form** is used to gather personal information such as the patient's name, address, employer, insurance company, and any known allergies. Every new patient must complete one of these forms on his or her initial visit. An established patient may also need to complete this form if any pertinent information such as employer, insurance carrier, or address needs to be updated.

> **HIPAA Tip >** The HIPAA Privacy Rule is the first comprehensive federal protection for the privacy of health information. These national standards protect individuals' medical records and other personal health information. The privacy rule must be followed by all health plans, health care clearinghouses, health care providers, and their business associates. The rules mandate that these groups must
>
> - Adopt privacy practices that are appropriate for their health care services
>
> - Notify patients about their privacy rights and how their information can be used or disclosed
>
> - Train employees so that they understand the privacy practices
>
> - Appoint a staff member to be the privacy official responsible for seeing that the privacy practices are adopted and followed
>
> - Secure patient records containing individually identifiable health information so that they are not readily available to those who do not need them

PATIENT INFORMATION FORM

THIS SECTION REFERS TO PATIENT ONLY

Name: Lisa Lomos	Sex: F	Marital Status: ☒S ☐M ☐D ☐W	Birth Date: 6/3/04

Address: 12 Briar Lane	SS#: 212-55-3311

City: Stephenson	State: OH	Zip: 60089	Employer:

Home Phone: 614-221-0202	Employer's Address:

Work Phone: 614-299-0313	City:	State:	Zip:

Spouse's Name:	Spouse's Employer:

Emergency Contact:	Relationship:	Phone #:

FILL IN IF PATIENT IS A MINOR

Parent/Guardian's Name: Juan Lomos	Sex: M	Marital Status: ☐S ☒M ☐D ☐W	Birth Date: 7/21/52

Phone: 614-221-0202	SS#: 716-83-0061

Address: 12 Briar Lane	Employer: Stephenson Wire Works

City: Stephenson	State: OH	Zip: 60089	Employer's Address: 125 Stephenson Road

Student Status: full-time	City: Stephenson	State: OH	Zip: 60089

INSURANCE INFORMATION

Primary Insurance Company: Blue Cross Blue Shield	Secondary Insurance Company: Physician's Alliance of Ohio

Subscriber's Name: Juan Lomos	Birth Date: 7/21/52	Rel. to Insured child	Subscriber's Name: Cedera Lomos	Birth Date: 5/21/57	Rel. to Insured child

Plan: Traditional	SS#: 716-83-0061	Plan: Traditional	SS#: 717-87-0054

Policy #: 716830061	Group #: 126	Policy #: 621382	Group #: A435

Copayment/Deductible: $250	Price Code: A	Copayment/Deductible: $100	Price Code: A

OTHER INFORMATION

Reason for visit: Routine well-child checkup	Allergy to Medication (list):

Name of referring physician:	If auto accident, list date and state in which it occurred:

Regardless of any insurance coverage I may or may not have, it is my responsibility to pay the entire bill. In the event that this office needs to obtain legal assistance in collection of any unpaid balance, I agree to pay costs and attorney fees, as allowable by law. I authorize the release of the above patient's medical records for billing purposes. I authorize payment of medical benefits to Dr. Katherine Yan, Dr. Jessica Rudner, or Dr. John Rudner.

Juan Lomos	9/4/09
(Patient's Signature/Parent or Guardian's Signature)	(Date)

Figure 4-1 *Sample Patient Information Form*

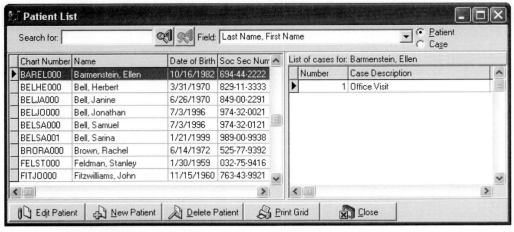

Figure 4-2   *Patient List Window*

Patient/Guarantor Information Requirements

As you can see by looking at Figure 4-1, the patient information form contains a substantial amount of information. Some of this information is used when you add a new patient to the patient database. The other information contained on the form is required when you set up a new case for a patient. You will learn how to perform both of these functions in this chapter.

The option to add a new patient is located in the Patient List window that appears when you choose Patients/Guarantors and Cases from the Lists menu (see Figure 4-2).

To enter a new patient in NDCMedisoft™, you click the New Patient button located at the bottom of the Patient List window. When this button is clicked, the Patient/Guarantor window is displayed (see Figure 4-3).

The following fields are listed in the Name/Address folder within the Patient/Guarantor window:

- Chart Number
- Patient Name (Last Name, First Name, and Middle Initial)
- Address (Street, City, State, ZIP Code, and Country)
- E-mail
- Phone Numbers (Home, Work, Cell, Fax, Other)
- Birth Date
- Sex
- Birth Weight and Units
- Social Security Number

The following fields are listed in the Other Information folder (see Figure 4-4):

- Type
- Assigned Provider
- Patient ID #2
- Patient Billing Code

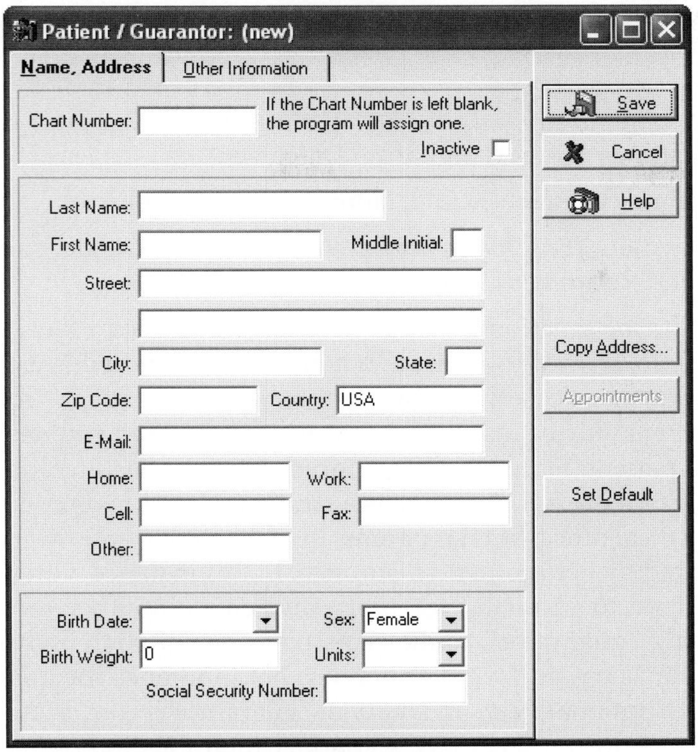

Figure 4-3   *Patient/Guarantor (New) Window*

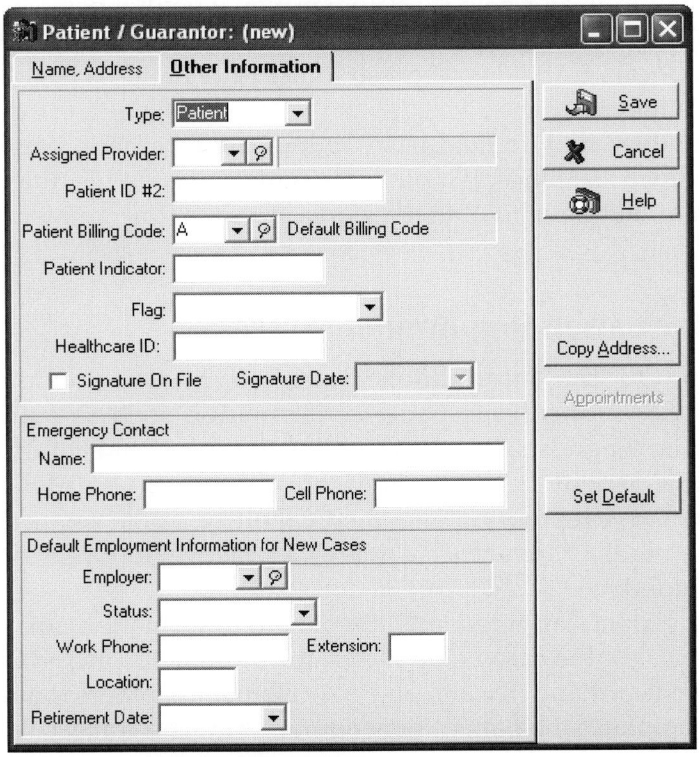

Figure 4-4   *Other Information Folder*

- Patient Indicator
- Flag
- Healthcare ID
- Signature on File and Signature Date
- Emergency Contact (Name, Home Phone, Cell Phone)
- Employment (Employer, Status, Work Phone and Extension, Location, and Retirement Date)

Most of the information is self-explanatory except for a few of the fields. The **Type** field is used to indicate whether an individual is a patient or a guarantor. In most cases, you will probably use "patient" for the type. However, there may be instances when the information you need to record is not for a patient. Suppose, for example, that you need to add a new patient account for Mary Lopez. She is a student who attends college in a city near the medical office, but her parents live in another state. Mary, however, is still covered by her mother's insurance. In this instance, you would need to set the type to "patient" for Mary and create another record for her mother using "guarantor" as the type. Later, when you enter the case information for Mary, you would reference her mother as the guarantor.

One of the optional fields in a patient/guarantor record is the Patient ID #2 field. This field can serve as a secondary identification code assigned to a patient or guarantor. The code can be displayed in lieu of a chart number on certain reports.

The **Patient Billing Code** field is also optional and may contain a user-defined one- or two-character entry that can be used to divide the practice into various groups for billing purposes.

The Patient Indicator field is another optional field. If desired, it can contain up to five characters that identify the patient for sorting purposes.

The Healthcare ID field is reserved for a future national health care identification number.

The **Signature on File** field lets you indicate whether a patient's signature is on file in the office. If a patient's signature is on file, the medical office staff may not have to obtain a signature each time an insurance claim is filed.

Case Information Requirements

In addition to the information described in the previous section, NDCMedisoft™ stores some patient information such as marital status, account data, diagnosis, insurance policy numbers, and condition in case records. The patient case data is organized into nine different folders. (See Figure 4-5.) Depending on a medical office's data requirements and the requirements of insurance carriers, a practice may not use all of the fields provided.

Using the data provided on the patient information form, you can complete most of the case fields except for those fields included in the Diagnosis, Medicaid and Tricare, and Miscellaneous folders. Later, after the provider completes the patient's encounter form, you can use it to enter the additional information.

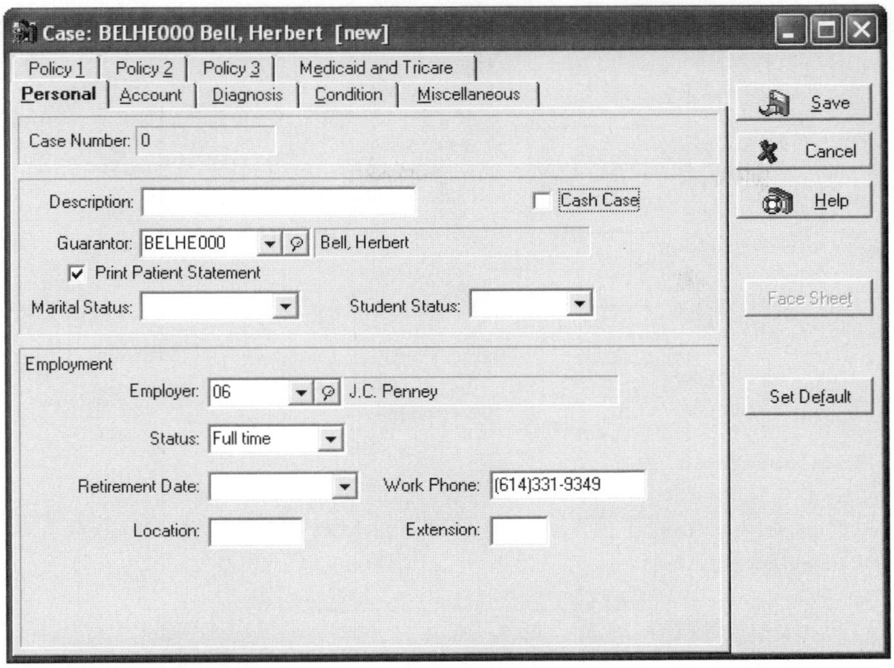

Figure 4-5 *Case Window*

An overview of the information needed to complete a patient case record is provided in the following paragraphs. Review this information before you continue with the practice exercises.

Personal The Personal folder (see Figure 4-5) contains personal data about a patient along with the case number, which is assigned automatically. When you complete this folder, you must enter a brief case description or reason for the visit. This folder also includes fields to enter the guarantor, marital status, student status, and employment information.

Account The Account folder, as shown in Figure 4-6 on page 62, holds pertinent information concerning the patient's account. Use this folder to record the assigned provider, referring provider, supervising provider, referral source, attorney, and facility codes. The codes needed to complete these fields must be set up in the Address file first.

The **case billing code,** which is included in the Account folder, lets you group or organize patients for billing purposes. How you use this code depends on the medical office's specific billing requirements. For example, you could assign billing code A to patients who will receive their bills on the fifteenth of the month and code B for patients billed on the thirtieth.

The price code determines which of the fee schedules is used to determine the amount charged for services. Each procedure code can have up to twenty-six different fees. The fees are listed in the Amounts tab of each procedure code entered in NDCMedisoft™.

Another part of the Account folder contains the visit series information. Some insurance companies may require the patient to receive authorization before seeking medical services. A carrier may also authorize only a specific

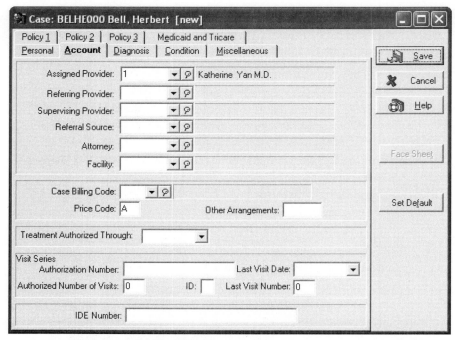

Figure 4-6   *Case Window (Account Folder)*

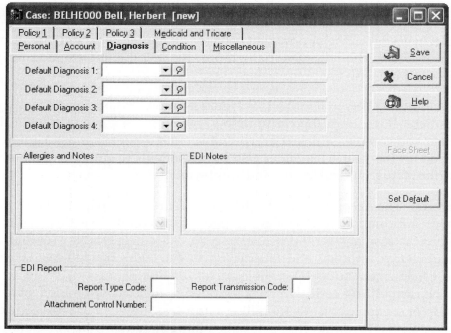

Figure 4-7   *Case Window (Diagnosis Folder)*

number of visits. In these instances, you can use this area to record the necessary information. The number "counts down" the number of allowed visits.

Diagnosis After a provider completes a patient's encounter form, you can use it to enter the diagnosis information in the Diagnosis folder (see Figure 4-7). You may enter up to four different diagnosis codes. As you may recall, these codes are stored in the Diagnosis database.

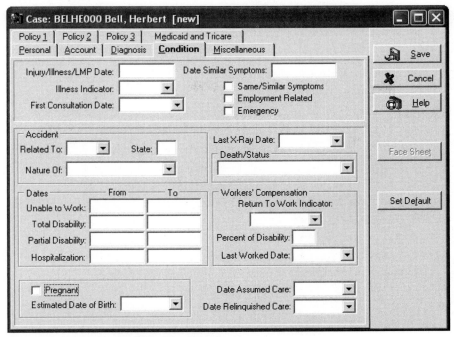

Figure 4-8   *Case Window (Condition Folder)*

The Diagnosis folder also provides space for you to indicate any allergies that the patient may have. The EDI Notes and Report fields are used to record specific information about the electronic claims for this particular case.

Condition You can store information related to a patient's illness or injury in the Condition folder (see Figure 4-8). In this folder, you can include data such as first consultation date, last X-ray date, and workers' compensation information.

Miscellaneous The Miscellaneous folder lets you indicate outside lab work and charges (see Figure 4-9 on page 64). There are other fields to record extra information about a patient. As with other fields in the case folders, these fields are optional.

Policy 1, Policy 2, and Policy 3 Although most patients have only one insurance policy, some patients have several different policies with varying coverage. For example, a retired person may have Medicare as her primary insurance. However, she may also have a supplemental policy to cover those expenses not reimbursed by Medicare.

Using the Policy folders, you can enter information for up to three different insurance policies. Most of the fields in the three folders are identical, except that Policy 1 asks for additional information, such copayment and deductible information (see Figure 4-10 on page 64). Some insurance policies have patients pay a copayment for each office visit or other service performed. The patient's insurance company pays the remainder of the bill directly to the provider. The **copayment** is a standard fee (usually $10 to $20) paid to the provider by a patient at the time of the appointment.

The Policy 1 Folder also contains a box to indicate whether the insurance plan is capitated. A **capitated plan** pays the provider a fixed amount

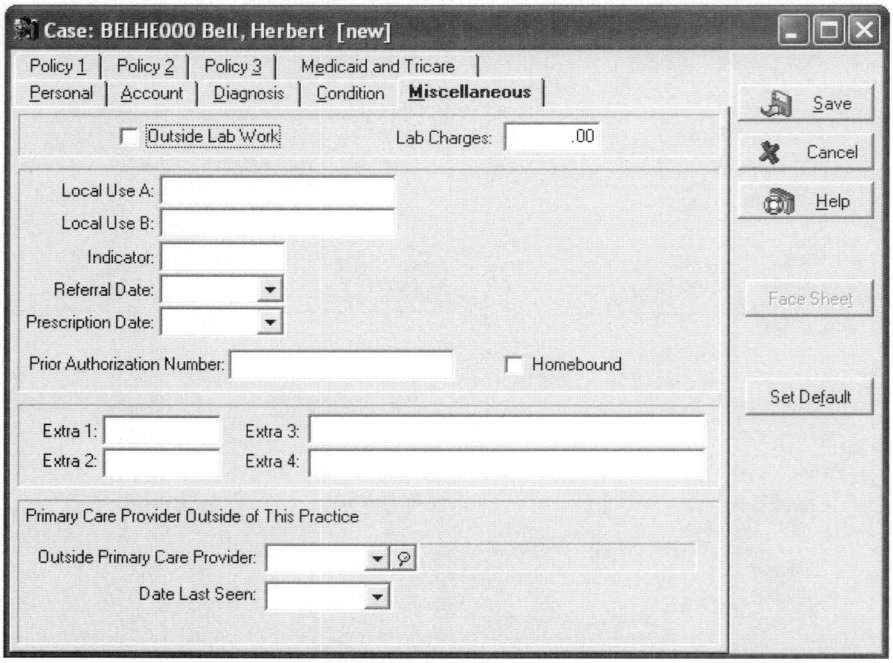

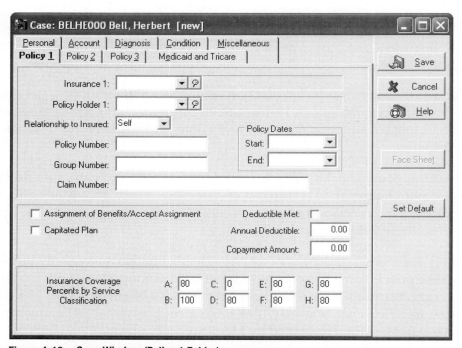

Figure 4-9 *Case Window (Miscellaneous Folder)*

Figure 4-10 *Case Window (Policy 1 Folder)*

regardless of whether the patient is or is not seen by the physician during the time period the payment covers. Many capitated plans pay providers this preset amount on a monthly basis.

For the second policy, you need to indicate whether there is automatic crossover between the two policies. For example, Medicare will automatically forward any unpaid portion of a claim to the secondary carrier. If the crossover is not facilitated by the primary carrier, the box should not be checked because the office will need to submit the claim to the secondary carrier.

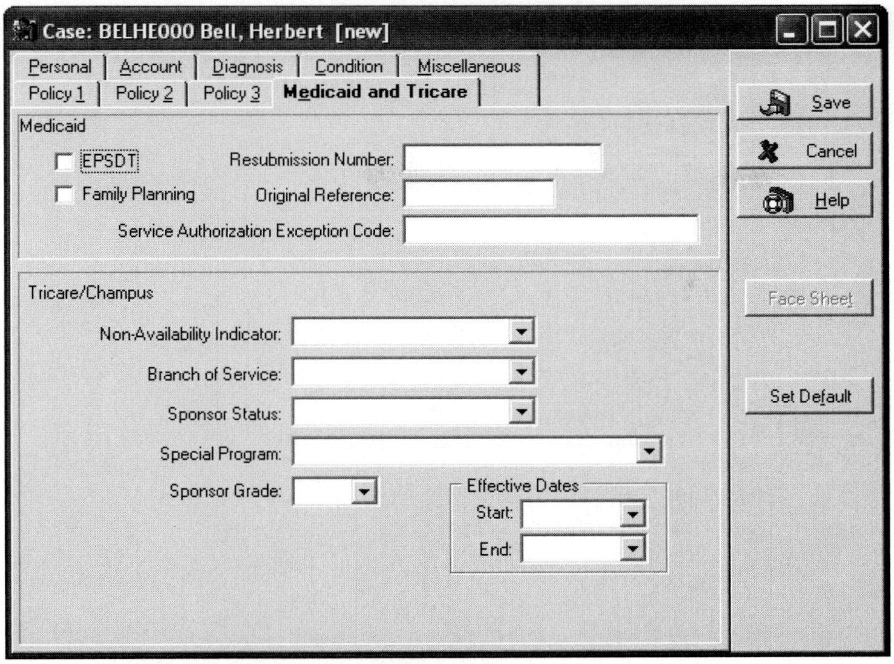

Figure 4-11 *Case Window (Medicaid and Tricare Folder)*

When you complete a patient's policy information, you must identify the policy holder and that individual's relationship to the patient. For a single person with his or her own policy, the policyholder is the patient, and the relationship to the insured is indicated as "self." Suppose that the patient is a child. In this instance, you would most likely identify a parent as the policyholder and the relationship as "child." Other important information needed to complete a Policy folder includes insurance carrier, assignment of benefits, policy number, group number, policy dates, and insurance coverage percentages.

Medicaid and Tricare Use the Medicaid and Tricare folder to record related information such as resubmission numbers, references, and effective dates (see Figure 4-11). For patients covered by Medicaid, you can also indicate whether additional coverage is provided by **EPSDT** (a well-baby program) or Family Planning. If a patient is covered by TRICARE, you can list the branch of service (such as Air Force, Army, Marines) and the sponsor status (such as 100 percent disabled, civilian, active duty).

✓CHECKPOINT

1. Which folder would you use to enter a brief description of a case?

2. When you enter a patient case, where should you record a patient's assigned provider or referring provider?

3. Is a patient's birth date required when you enter a new case? If not, where do you enter this information?

4. Where do you enter a patient's Social Security number?

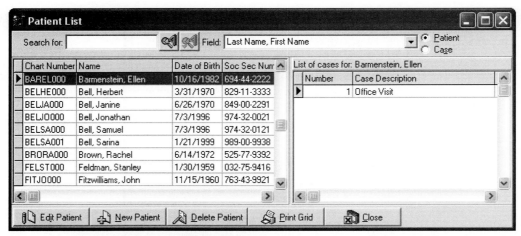

Figure 4-12   *Patient List Window with Patient Selected*

Entering Patient and Case Data

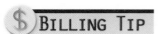

> ## $BILLING TIP
>
> *You can use the Patient/ Case radio buttons to set the active area of the window, or use your mouse to click anywhere in the desired list to make it active.*

NDCMedisoft™ makes it easy to enter a new patient record, edit existing data, or delete a patient record. Once you add a new patient to the patient file, filling in the case information is also a straightforward process.

To enter the information you read about in this chapter, use the Patients/ Guarantors and Cases option in the Lists menu. When you choose this option, the NDCMedisoft™ program displays the Patient List window. As shown in Figures 4-12 and 4-13, the patient list appears on the left side of the window, and the case list appears on the right side of the window. The radio buttons (Patient, Case) at the top right corner of the window indicate the current focus. When the patient list is active, as shown in Figure 4-12, the Edit Patient, New Patient, and Delete Patient buttons appear at the bottom of the window. When the case list is active, as shown in Figure 4-13, the Edit Case, New Case, Delete Case, and Copy Case buttons are displayed.

To begin adding a new patient to the data file, you would click the New Patient button. If you need to edit or delete a patient record, first select the desired patient, and then click the corresponding button. You can select a patient record by searching or by scrolling through the list and clicking a patient's chart number.

The case records that appear on the right side of the Patient List window are linked to the selected patient. Only those cases entered for the selected patient appear in the list. Remember that you must click the button for the Case list before the program displays the cases.

To work with patient case records, first locate and select a patient record. Then click the New Case button to add a new case for that patient. To save time, you can highlight an existing case and click the Copy Case button to make a copy of a case record. Then just make the necessary changes. When you need to edit or delete a case, select it and then click the appropriate button.

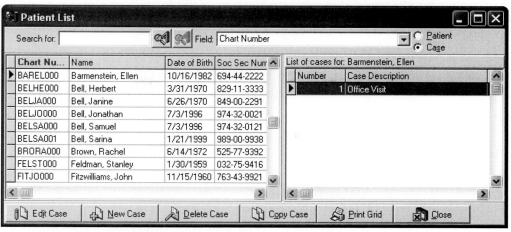

Figure 4-13 *Patient List Window with Case Selected*

✓CHECKPOINT

5. Which menu option should you choose to add a new patient record?

6. Which button can you choose to duplicate an existing case?

7. Does the NDCMedisoft™ program automatically assign a case number? Can you set it manually?

8. Which button in the Patient List window lets you change a patient's address?

Computer Practice 4-1: *Adding a New Patient and Case Record (Juan Lomos)*

Follow these steps to add a new patient and case record:

1. Start the NDCMedisoft™ software.

2. Set the program date to September 4, 2009.

3. Restore the backup file that you created at the end of Chapter 3.

4. Select the Patients/Guarantors and Cases option from the Lists menu, or use the toolbar to select this option (Patient List button). When you choose this option, the Patient List window appears.

5. Juan Lomos, a new patient, completed the patient information form (Source Document 1). Review the information provided on the form.

6. To add a new patient, click the New Patient button provided in the Patient List window.

7. Using the information on Source Document 1, enter the patient's name, address, phone numbers, birth date, gender, and Social Security number in the Name, Address folder. Note: You don't

$ BILLING TIP

• Make sure the patient list is selected. Check the radio buttons at the top of the window.

• When you enter a phone number, don't enter the parentheses or the hyphen. Just enter the numbers, such as 6142210202. The program automatically formats the phone number. The same is true for the Social Security number. Enter the birth date as 07211952—the program adds slashes for you.

need to enter a chart number; the NDCMedisoft™ program will automatically assign this number.

8. Switch to the Other Information folder.

9. Verify that the Type field is set to Patient, and select the assigned provider, Dr. Katherine Yan, in the Assigned Provider box.

10. Verify that the Patient Billing Code is set to A.

11. Click the Signature on File box, and enter the date of the office visit in the Signature Date box. After you enter the date, a Confirm box appears, notifying you that you have entered a date that is in the future, and asking whether you want to change it. Click the No button. A Warning box appears, reminding you that the Signature on File date that you entered is in the future. Click the OK button. (Note: These Confirm and Warning boxes will appear when you enter dates in the program, because the dates being used for the exercises are set in 2009.)

12. Click on the Employer drop-down list button. As you can see, Juan's employer, Stephenson Wire Works, is not listed. You need to add his employer to the Address list before you can continue.

13. Place the cursor in the Employer box, and press the F8 key. (Or you may choose the Addresses option from the Lists menu, and then click the New button.)

14. Enter the address information for Stephenson Wire Works in the Address window. Use 15 for the employer code. Click the Save button in the Address window to save this new record. Close the Address List window, if necessary.

15. Now you can complete the employer information (code, status, and work phone).

16. Review the information you entered in the Name, Address and Other Information folders. If you notice a mistake, correct the error.

17. Click the Save button to save the new patient information. The program will assign the chart number when it saves the record.

18. Locate the new record you just added. It should be the selected patient in the Patient List window. If Juan Lomos is not selected, click on his record to select it.

19. Click the Case radio button or click on the right side of the Patient List window so that you can enter the case information for Juan Lomos.

20. Click the New Case button.

21. In the Personal folder, enter the following information from Source Document 1: case description, guarantor, and marital status. Use the information written on the source document in the Reason for Visit field to complete the Description field in the data entry window. As shown on Juan's patient information form, he is the insurance policyholder. Therefore, this also makes him the

guarantor. The employment information should already be included in the folder.

22. Switch to the Account folder. Several of the fields should already contain data that the NDCMedisoft™ program gathers from other databases. Verify the price code from Source Document 1.

23. Select the Condition folder.

24. Since Juan's visit was due to an automobile accident, you need to enter this information in the Condition folder. Enter the accident date (8/8/09) in the Injury/Illness/LMP (Last Menstrual Period) Date field. Place a check in the Emergency box, since this was an emergency. Set the Accident, Related To field to Auto and enter *OH* in the Accident, State field.

25. Use the additional information prepared by Dr. Yan (Source Document 2) to complete the Total Disability, Partial Disability, and Hospitalization date fields in the Condition folder.

26. Select the Policy 1 folder.

27. Enter Juan's primary insurance carrier (Blue Cross/Blue Shield) in the Insurance 1 box.

28. Verify that Juan's chart number is selected to indicate that he is the policyholder and that the Relationship to Insured box is set to Self.

29. Record Juan's policy number (716830061) and group number (126).

30. Click the Assignment of Benefits/Accept Assignment box so that an *X* appears in the box.

31. Enter Juan's deductible amount ($250.00) in the Annual Deductible box. Since Juan has met his deductible for 2009, place a check in the Deductible Met box.

32. Enter *80* in each of the Insurance Coverage Percents by Service Classification boxes, since Juan's insurance pays 80 percent of covered charges.

33. Review the information you entered in each of the folders. Make any needed corrections.

34. Save the case information. When you click the Save button, the NDCMedisoft™ program will automatically assign a case number.

35. Verify that a case record for Juan Lomos appears in the Patient List window.

Computer Practice 4-2: *Adding a New Patient (Cedera Lomos)*

Follow the steps provided here to add a new patient and case record for Juan Lomos' wife, Cedera. Cedera is also a new patient of Dr. Katherine Yan. Review the information she recorded on the patient information form (Source Document 3.)

1. Click the New Patient button to begin entering the new patient information for Cedera Lomos.

2. From the patient information form that Cedera completed (Source Document 3), enter the information in the Name, Address and Other Information folders. For this patient, and each time you add a new patient, be sure to complete the Signature on File and Signature Date fields using the date of the office visit.

3. Review the information you entered, correct any errors, and save the new patient record.

4. Click the Case button and then click the New Case button to add a case for Cedera Lomos.

5. Complete the case folders as follows.

   - Enter the information for the Personal folder. Since Cedera indicated that her husband's insurance is the primary policy, make sure that you select Juan Lomos as the guarantor.

   - Enter any necessary information in the Account folder.

   - Make a note of Cedera's allergy to penicillin. Enter this information in the Diagnosis folder.

   - Enter the primary insurance information in the Policy 1 folder. Be sure to enter Juan Lomos as the policyholder and enter Spouse in the Relationship to Insured field. Select Blue Cross/Blue Shield for the insurance, and enter the other pertinent data.

   - Record the secondary insurance information in the Policy 2 folder. In this instance, Cedera is the insured party and the relationship is "self." Enter the insurance company (Physician's Alliance of Ohio), policy number (621382), the group number (A435), and click the Assignment of Benefits box. Enter *80* in the Insurance Coverage boxes at the bottom of the Policy 2 folder.

6. Review your work, and then save the case data.

Computer Practice 4-3: *Adding a New Patient (Lisa Lomos)*

Follow steps similar to those listed above to add a new patient and case record for Juan and Cedera Lomos' daughter, Lisa (also a patient of Dr. Yan). Review the information recorded on her patient information form (Source Document 4.)

1. Record the patient information for Lisa Lomos.

2. Review your work, and save the patient data.

3. Complete the case information that is shown on Lisa's patient information form.

4. Check the information you entered, and save the new case record.

Computer Practice 4-4: *Adding a New Patient (Angela Wong)*

Follow the steps you learned in the previous practice exercises to add a new patient record and case for Angela Wong (also a patient of Dr. Yan). Review the information she recorded on the patient information form (Source Document 5.)

IMPORTANT: Angela is a full-time student who is covered by her father's insurance. Her father, Peter Wong, is the guarantor and the insured party. Since her father is not a patient at the Family Care Center, you will have to enter him as a guarantor before you can complete the case information for Angela. The steps to add a guarantor are the same as those for adding a new patient. For the Type field in the Other Information folder, choose Guarantor instead of Patient for Peter Wong. In Angela's Policy 1 folder, be sure to click the Assignment of Benefits box and enter the copayment amount, which is $10. Enter *100* in each of the Insurance Coverage boxes at the bottom of the Policy 1 folder.

Computer Practice 4-5: *Editing a Patient Record (John Fitzwilliams)*

An existing patient, John Fitzwilliams, changed jobs. Previously, he was self-employed. Review the information on Source Document 6. Then follow these steps to edit Mr. Fitzwilliams's patient record.

1. Select the Patients/Guarantors and Cases option from the Lists menu if the Patient List window is not displayed, or use the toolbar to select this option.

2. Make sure the patient list (left side of the window) is active.

3. Use the Search feature or scroll through the patient list to select John Fitzwilliams's record.

4. Click the Edit Patient button to edit the patient's data.

5. Switch to the Other Information folder.

6. Change the employment information as indicated on Source Document 6.

7. Save the changes you made.

> **$ BILLING TIP**
>
> *If a case record existed for this patient, you would also need to change the employment information in the Personal folder of the Case window.*

> **$ BILLING TIP**
>
> *As a shortcut, you can double-click on a case or patient record to edit it.*

Computer Practice 4-6: *Updating Case Information (Herbert Mitchell)*

Follow these steps to update the case information for Herbert Mitchell (see Source Document 7.)

1. Select the Patients/Guarantors and Cases option from the Lists menu if the Patient List window is not displayed.

2. Make sure the patient list (left side of the window) is in focus.

3. Use the Search feature or scroll through the patient list to select Mr. Mitchell's record.

4. Once you locate and select his record, select the Shortness of Breath case by clicking on it.

5. Click the Edit Case button so that you can update the case information.

6. Choose the Condition folder, and enter the hospitalization dates shown on Source Document 7.

7. Enter the Medicare authorization number in the Miscellaneous folder.

8. Save the changes you made.

9. Close the Patient List window.

Computer Practice 4-7: *Exiting the Program and Making a Backup Copy*

Practice quitting the software and making a backup copy of your work by following these steps:

1. Choose Exit from the File menu, or use the toolbar to select this option.

2. Insert your working copy of the Student Data Disk in Drive A:

3. Click the Back Up Data Now button.

4. In the Destination File Path and Name box, enter *A:\PBChap4.mbk,* where A represents the drive where you are saving your work.

5. Click the Start Backup button. When the Backup Complete box appears, click OK. The NDCMedisoft™ program shuts down.

6. Remove the floppy disk from Drive A:.

7. Store your disk in a safe place.

Chapter 4 Review

Define the Terms

Write a definition for each term: (Obj. 4-1)

1. Capitated plan

   _____

2. Case billing code

   _____

3. Copayment

   _____

4. EPSDT

   _____

5. Established patient

   _____

6. New patient

   _____

7. Patient billing code

   _____

8. Patient information form

   _____

9. Signature on file

   _____

10. Type

   _____

Check Your Understanding

11. Which folders in the Case window do you use to enter the insurance information? (Obj. 4-4)

   _____

12. Where do you indicate whether an individual is a patient or a guarantor? Describe a situation where a person would need to be entered into the system as a guarantor, but not as a patient. Can a patient also be a guarantor? Explain. (Obj. 4-2)

_____

_____

_____

13. What is the Patient ID #2 field? How can it be used? (Obj. 4-3)

_____

_____

14. What information is recorded in the Personal folder of a case record? (Obj. 4-4)

_____

_____

15. Where would you record a patient's allergy to a prescription drug such as penicillin? (Obj. 4-4)

_____

16. A patient has Blue Cross and Blue Shield insurance coverage through her employer. She is also covered under her husband's Prudential policy for expenses that Blue Cross and Blue Shield does not cover. How do you enter information on her insurance? (Obj. 4-5)

_____

_____

CRITICAL ANALYSIS EXERCISE

17. A patient has been seen by the physician for hypertension on several occasions within the past six months. The physician just received a phone call from the patient's wife, stating that the patient is experiencing palpitations and dizziness. The physician suggests taking the patient to the emergency room at the local hospital, where the physician will meet the patient and his wife. Would you need to create a new case? Do you have enough information to make the decision? If not, what additional information would you need? (Obj. 4-4)

_____

_____

_____

Processing Transactions

WHAT YOU NEED TO KNOW

To complete this chapter, you need to know how to:

- Enter information in NDCMedisoft™.
- Navigate the NDCMedisoft™ software.
- Search for information in an NDCMedisoft™ database.
- Enter patient and case information.

WHAT YOU WILL LEARN

When you finish this chapter, you will be able to:

1. Define the terms introduced in this chapter.
2. Explain the information contained on a patient's encounter form and how it is used to record a transaction.
3. Enter procedure charge transactions.
4. Record and apply payments received from patients and insurance carriers.
5. Print a walkout receipt.
6. Enter an adjustment.

KEY TERMS

Adjustment An amount, positive or negative, entered to correct a patient's account balance.

Charge The amount (or cost) of a procedure performed by a provider.

Default An entry automatically displayed in an input field (can be overwritten).

Inpatient Refers to a patient admitted to a hospital who stays there for one or more days before being discharged.

Insurance payments Payments made to the practice by insurance carriers.

Modifiers One- or two-digit codes that allow more specific descriptions to be entered for the services the physician performed.

MultiLink code A code that incorporates a number of individual procedure codes that are related.

Outpatient Refers to a patient who is treated at a hospital but does not stay overnight.

Patient payments Cash, checks, or credit card charges from patients for services rendered.

Remittance advice (RA) A document received from an insurance carrier that lists patients, dates of service, charges, and the amounts paid and denied.

Handling Transactions

During a typical day, many patients visit a medical practice such as the Family Care Center. For each patient, the assigned provider will perform specific procedures related to that patient's condition. The physician records the procedures performed on each patient's encounter form. In turn, the billing assistant uses the completed encounter form as a source document to enter the procedure charge(s). A **charge** is the cost that a medical office assigns to a procedure.

A billing assistant must process payments on a daily basis. Insurance companies send payments for covered procedures on behalf of patients. These payments are transmitted electronically or mailed to the practice. Some patients make copayments at the time of a visit. Others send their payments by mail later, after insurance company payments have been received.

On occasion, it may be necessary to make an adjustment to a patient's account. An **adjustment** is an amount (positive or negative) entered to correct a patient's account balance. An adjustment might be required, for example, if an insurance company did not pay as much as expected.

As you will learn in this chapter, the NDCMedisoft™ program can be used to process several different kinds of transactions—charges, payments, and adjustments. First, you will learn how to record and enter procedure charges. Then you will learn how to process payments and adjustments.

Recording and Entering Procedure Charges

For every procedure performed, a billing assistant must make sure that the appropriate information is properly recorded in the patient accounting system. Recording the procedure charges properly is an important first step in the billing cycle. Activities such as managing cash flow, collecting payments, processing claims, and generating reports all depend on this first step.

Reviewing a Completed Encounter Form

As you learned in a previous chapter, the completed encounter form is the primary source of information that a billing assistant needs to record procedure charges. As shown in Figure 5-1, this completed encounter form includes the following information: provider's name, patient's name and

9/4/09	**Family Care Center**	**Dr. Katherine Yan**
DATE	**285 Stephenson Boulevard**	PROVIDER
Hiro Tanaka	**Stephenson, OH 60089**	**TANHIO00**
PATIENT NAME	**614-555-0100**	CHART #

OFFICE VISITS - SYMPTOMATIC	
99201	OF--New Patient Minimal
99202	OF--New Patient Low
99203	OF--New Patient Detailed
99204	OF--New Patient Moderate
99205	OF--New Patient High
99211	OF--Established Patient Minimal
99212	OF--Established Patient Low
99213	OF--Established Patient Detailed
99214	OF--Established Patient Moderate
99215	OF--Established Patient High
PREVENTIVE VISITS	
NEW	
99381	Under 1 Year
99382	1 - 4 Years
99383	5 - 11 Years
99384	12 - 17 Years
99385	18 - 39 Years
99386	40 - 64 Years
99387	65 Years & Up
ESTABLISHED	
99391	Under 1 Year
99392	1 - 4 Years
99393	5 - 11 Years
99394	12 - 17 Years
99395	18 - 39 Years
99396	40 - 64 Years
99397	65 Years & Up
PROCEDURES	
12011	Repair of superficial wounds, face
29125	Short arm splint
45378	Colonoscopy--diagnostic
45380	Colonoscopy--biopsy
71010	Chest x-ray, frontal
71020	Chest x-ray, frontal and lateral
73070	Elbow x-ray, AP and lateral

73090	Forearm x-ray, AP and lateral
73100	Wrist x-ray, AP and lateral
PROCEDURES	
73600	Ankle x-ray, AP and lateral
93000	Electrocardiogram--EEG
93015	Treadmill stress test
LABORATORY	
80061	Lipid panel
82270	Hemoccult--stool screening
82465	Cholesterol test
82947	Glucose--quantitative
82951	Glucose tolerance test
83718	HDL cholesterol test
85007	Manual WBC
85025	CBC w/diff.
85651	Erythrocyte sed rate--ESR
86585	Tine test
87040	Strep culture
87430	Strep screen
87086	Urine colony count
87088	Urine culture
INJECTIONS	
90471	Immunization administration
90657	Influenza injection, under 35 months
90658	Influenza injection, older than 3 years
90703	Tetanus immunization
90707	MMR immunization

REFERRING PHYSICIAN	NPI	NOTES
AUTHORIZATION #		
DIAGNOSIS **848.9**		
PAYMENT AMOUNT **$10 copayment, check #3022**		

Figure 5-1 *Completed Encounter Form*

chart number, date the services were performed, procedures performed, payments received, diagnosis, and other information.

After a physician completes a patient examination, he or she will mark the procedures performed. As you may recall, the encounter form includes only the most common procedures provided by a medical office. If the physician performs a procedure not listed on the encounter form, he or she writes the procedure in on the form. In these instances, you will have to search for and enter the procedure code when processing a charge.

Most insurance carriers will not pay for treatment without a diagnosis. The diagnosis is the doctor's opinion of a patient's condition. Therefore, the doctor must record this information on the encounter form so that it can be included as part of the procedure charge. When you enter the diagnosis, you will use the ICD-9 codes as a standard way to record this information.

Entering a Procedure Charge

After you review a patient's encounter form, you are ready to enter the transaction to record the procedure charge. You will process all charge transactions using the Enter Transactions option in the Activities menu. Selecting this option displays the Transaction Entry window. As you can see in Figure 5-2, transactions are case-based. That is, every transaction, including charges, must be assigned to a patient and a specific case. You cannot enter or edit a transaction until you select a chart number and a case number.

When you enter procedure charges, you must enter a separate transaction for each charge rather than combining all procedures into a single

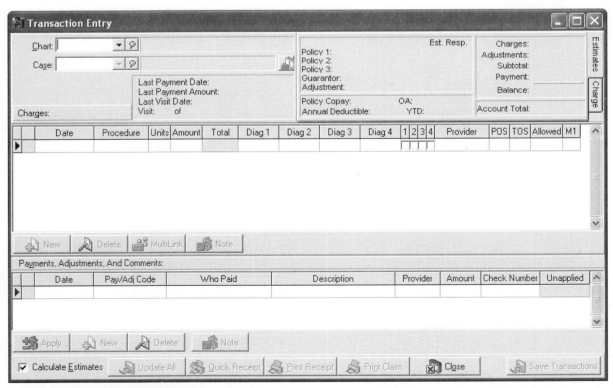

Figure 5-2 *Transaction Entry Dialog Box*

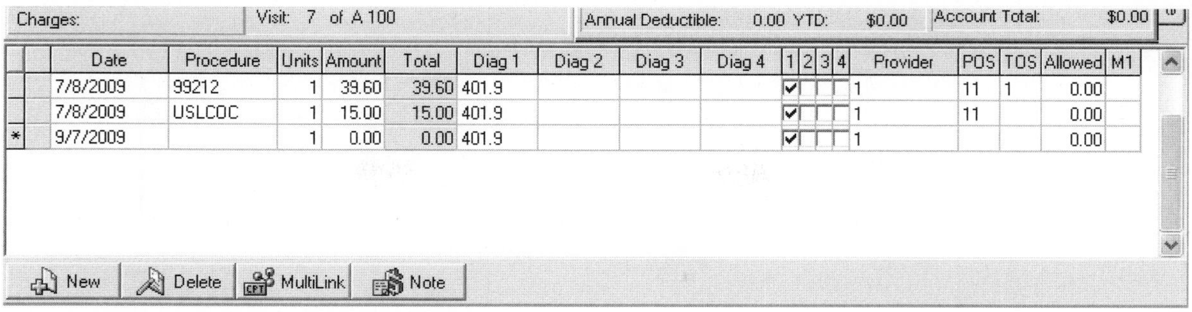

Figure 5-3 *Charges Area within the Transaction Entry Dialog Box*

transaction. This step is required because you must provide detailed information about each charge, including a description and an amount.

Once you enter a chart number and a case number, you can choose to enter a new transaction by clicking the New button in the Charges section of the dialog box (see Figure 5-3). When you click this button, the program creates a new transaction line. A **default** is an entry that automatically appears in a field and will be accepted unless you change the information. By default, the program enters the current date (the NDCMedisoft™ Program Date) and other select information for the new transaction. Usually you do not have to change the default entries.

To record a procedure charge, you must identify the procedure by using its corresponding CPT code. When you enter a procedure code, the NDCMedisoft™ program automatically fills in the fields based on the information stored in the Procedure data file. This information can be edited if necessary.

After you record a procedure code, you can enter additional information in the M1 (Modifier 1) field to further define a procedure. **Modifiers** are one- or two-digit codes that allow more specific descriptions to be entered for the services the physician performed. For example, a modifier needs to be used when the circumstances require services beyond those normally associated with a particular procedure code. A common modifier is -90, which indicates that the procedure is performed by an outside laboratory. If a modifier is indicated on an encounter form, it is entered in the Modifier box—M1. Fields for entering up to three additional modifiers can be added if required.

Although most procedures take place in the office, some patients may receive inpatient or outpatient care. **Inpatient** refers to care provided when patients must stay overnight at a hospital. **Outpatient,** on the other hand, refers to medical care provided at a hospital when the patient does not stay overnight. Use the POS (place of service) field to enter a code that identifies the location for the procedure. These standard numerical codes are used:

11   Provider's office
21   Inpatient hospital
22   Outpatient hospital
23   Hospital emergency room

The Diag 1, 2, 3, and 4 boxes and the Diagnosis check boxes are used to link a procedure to a particular diagnosis. If a diagnosis has been entered in the Diagnosis tab of the Case folder, it will also appear here.

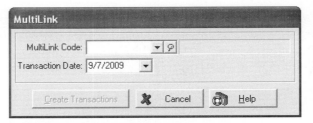

Figure 5-4 *MultiLink Dialog Box*

NDCMedisoft™ provides a feature that saves time when entering multiple CPT codes that are related. A **MultiLink code** is a single code that incorporates a number of procedure codes that relate to a single activity. Using MultiLink codes saves time by eliminating the need to enter related multiple procedure codes one at a time.

For example, suppose a MultiLink code is created for the procedures related to diagnosing strep throat. The code is labeled "STREP," and includes three procedures: 99212 Office Visit, Low; 87430 Strep screen; and 85025 CBC w/diff. When the MultiLink code STREP is selected, all three procedure codes are automatically entered by the system, eliminating the need to make three different entries. The MultiLink feature saves time by reducing the number of procedure code entries, and it also reduces omission errors. When procedure codes are entered as a MultiLink, it is impossible to forget to enter a procedure, since all of the codes that are in the MultiLink group are entered automatically.

Clicking the MultiLink button in the Transaction Entry dialog box displays the MultiLink dialog box (see Figure 5-4). After a MultiLink code is selected from the drop-down list, the Create Transactions button is clicked. The codes and charges for each procedure are automatically added to the list of transactions in the Transaction Entry dialog box.

Once you record the required information, the last step is to save the information you entered. Then, if there is another procedure charge, you repeat the same steps. After you record the last procedure, you can review the transaction data provided in the Estimates area in the top right corner of the dialog box. The Estimates area includes the procedure charge total, adjustments, payments, and account total. Information is also included regarding the estimated amount to be paid by the patient's insurance company.

Computer Practice 5-1: *Entering a Patient Charge Transaction (Cedera Lomos)*

The encounter form for Cedera Lomos is shown in Source Document 8. Record the procedure charge and the diagnosis by following these steps:

1. Start the NDCMedisoft™ program.

2. Set the program date to September 4, 2009.

3. Restore the backup file that you created at the end of Chapter 4.

4. Review the information shown on the encounter form in Source Document 8. As you can see, there is one procedure charge (OF—New Patient, Moderate) and a diagnosis (473.9) written on the encounter form.

5. Click Patients/Guarantors and Cases on the Lists menu. Enter *L* in the Search For box. Notice that the list of patients is reduced to those with chart numbers beginning with the letter *L*. With the Cedera Lomos line selected, click Persistent cough in the Case section of the window. Then click the Edit Case button.

6. Select the Diagnosis folder, and enter the diagnosis code from the encounter form in the Default Diagnosis 1 box. Then click the Save button.

7. Close the Patient List window, and select the Enter Transactions option from the Activities menu, or use the toolbar to select this option. When you choose this option, the Transaction Entry window appears.

8. In the Transaction Entry window, select Cedera's chart number, and then choose the case number for this visit. An Information window appears, reminding you that Cedera is allergic to penicillin. Click the OK button.

9. Click the New button in the Charges section of the dialog box to begin entering the procedure charge for Cedera Lomos.

10. Accept the default information shown in the date field. The date should be September 4, 2009.

11. Enter the procedure code (99204) for OF—New Patient, Moderate—in the Procedure field. Notice that the charge amount ($147.00) is automatically filled in when you enter the procedure code and press Tab.

12. Review the information in the other fields:
    - Accept 1 for the units.
    - Verify that the Amount field is set to $147.00. If not, first check that you entered the procedure code correctly. If it is correct, accept the amount.
    - For each charge, you need to identify a corresponding diagnosis. Since there was only one diagnosis, the program automatically selects it. Verify that the first Diagnosis check box is selected.
    - Accept the provider information. This field should already include the provider code for Dr. Yan.
    - Accept the information in the POS (place of service) field. The code should be set to 11, since this is the default code.
    - Accept the information in the TOS (type of service) field. Code 1 (medical care) is the default code for this field.

13. Click the Save Transactions button to save your work. A Date of Service Validation window will appear, reminding you that you

have entered a future date. In response to the question about saving the transaction, click the Yes button. (You will see this window whenever you save a transaction in this text, as the exercises take place in the future.)

14. When you save a transaction, the NDCMedisoft™ program updates the information (policy, charges, payments, last visit, and account total) shown in the top portion of the Transaction Entry screen. (See Figure 5-5.)

15. Close the Transaction Entry window.

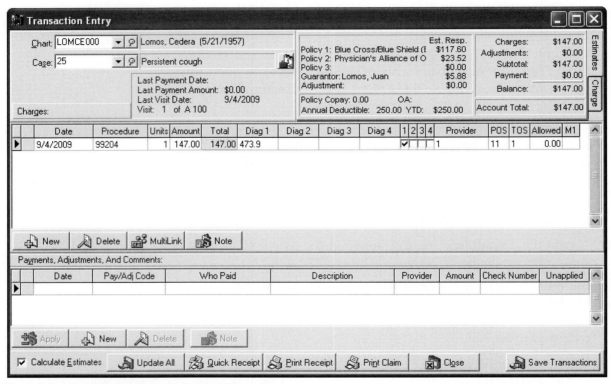

Figure 5-5   *Saved Transaction with Updated Information*

Computer Practice 5-2: *Entering a Patient Charge Transaction (Lisa Lomos)*

Record the procedure charge information for Lisa Lomos. The encounter form completed by Dr. Yan is shown in Source Document 9. As you can see, three procedures and two diagnoses are marked on this encounter form. The v20.2 (health checkup, infant or child) diagnosis is linked to the preventive procedure. The v06.4 (immunization—comb. of disease—MMR) diagnosis is linked to the injection and the MMR (measles, mumps, and rubella) procedures.

1. The date is still September 4, 2009. Select Patients/Guarantors and Cases from the Lists menu.

2. Select the chart number for Lisa Lomos, and open the case for her well-child checkup.

3. Click on the Diagnosis tab. Enter the v20.2 diagnosis as Default Diagnosis 1. Enter the other diagnosis as Default Diagnosis 2. Click the Save button.

4. Close the Patient List dialog box, and then select the Enter Transactions option from the Activities menu.

5. Select the chart number for Lisa Lomos, and verify that the well-child checkup case is selected.

6. Click the New button in the Charges section to record a new charge transaction.

7. Enter the charges from the encounter form. Leave the other default fields as they are unless you have specific information to change them.

8. Save the charge transactions.

9. Check your work. The account total should be $255.00 for Lisa Lomos.

Computer Practice 5-3: *Entering a Patient Charge and Adding a New Case and Insurance Carrier (Leila Patterson)*

Review the encounter form for Leila Patterson shown in Source Document 10. Leila is an established patient who made an appointment to have her cholesterol checked. During the office visit, Dr. Yan performed two procedures for this patient, both of which are linked to the one diagnosis. Note: Ms. Patterson has changed insurance carriers, so she has completed a new patient information form (Source Document 11). Her new carrier is not in the database, so you will need to enter it based on the information on Source Documents 11 and 12.

Follow the steps below to enter a patient charge. You will create a new case and add an insurance carrier in the process.

1. Verify that the NDCMedisoft™ Program Date is set to September 4, 2009.

2. Select Leila Patterson's chart number in the Transaction Entry window. When you do so, a default case code does not appear since there are no case records entered for Leila.

3. Move to the Case field.

4. As a shortcut, press the F8 function key to begin entering a new case. Another way to enter a new case would be to use the Patients/Guarantors and Cases option in the Lists menu, but the shortcut is much faster.

5. Complete the Description field in the Personal case folder.

6. Verify that A is listed in the Price Code field in the Account tab.

7. Enter the diagnosis in the Diagnosis tab.

8. Click the Policy 1 tab. When you try to select Patterson's insurance carrier, Oxford, you realize it is not in the list of carriers. To add Oxford to the database, use the F8 shortcut key to display the Insurance Carrier (new) dialog box. Use the information on Source Document 12 to complete the tabs. In the EDI, Codes tab, create the Default Payment Application codes at the bottom of the dialog box. Click in each box, and press F8 to display the Procedure/Payment/Adjustment (new) dialog box. The codes should be named as follows:

OXFPAY	Oxford Payment
OXFADJ	Oxford Adjustment
OXFWIT	Oxford Withhold
OXFDED	Oxford Deductible
OXFTAK	Oxford Take Back

Before you can complete the PINS tab, you must save the data on the new insurance carrier. When the Insurance Carrier dialog box for Oxford closes, you can open it again by clicking Insurance Carriers on the Lists menu, selecting the Oxford entry, and then clicking the Edit button. When you have finished your entries in the PINS tab, save your work, and close the Insurance Carrier List dialog box.

9. Back in the Policy 1 tab, you can now select Oxford from the list of insurance carriers. Fill in the other information in the Policy 1 tab using Source Documents 11 and 12. Dr. Yan does accept assignment for Oxford patients, so be sure to check that box. Also be sure to complete the Insurance Coverage Percents at the bottom of the dialog box. Oxford pays 80 percent of covered services.

10. Complete the new case entry by clicking the Save button.

11. In the Transaction Entry dialog box, enter both procedure charge transactions, and save your work. Accept the defaults for the information not provided on the encounter form. Ms. Patterson's account total should be $65.00.

Computer Practice 5-4: *Entering a Patient Charge and Adding a New Case (Ellen Barmenstein)*

Review the encounter form for Ellen Barmenstein shown in Source Document 13. Follow these steps to record her transactions.

1. Verify that the NDCMedisoft™ Program Date is set to September 4, 2009.

2. Select Ellen Barmenstein's chart number in the Transaction Entry window.

3. A case number appears, but today's visit is for another reason. Create a new case for this office visit. Enter a description in the Personal folder. Enter the diagnosis listed on the encounter form.

In the Policy 1 folder, enter Ms. Barmenstein as the policyholder. She is covered by Blue Cross/Blue Shield (policy: 13056; group: K1047; accept assignment: yes; annual deductible: 250; insurance coverage percents A-H: 80). Save the case information.

4. Enter the procedure charges.

5. Save your work. Barmenstein's account total should be $96.00. This includes unpaid charges from her August 29 visit. Her case balance should be $52.00.

6. Close the Transaction Entry dialog box.

✓CHECKPOINT

1. Which application menu option do you use to enter a procedure charge?

2. What document is the primary source of information that is used to record a procedure charge transaction?

3. What two pieces of information must be entered before you can enter a procedure charge?

Entering Payments

The next step is the processing of payments received from patients and insurance companies. Payments are entered in two different areas of the NDCMedisoft™ program: the Transaction Entry dialog box and the Deposit List dialog box. Practices may have different preferences for how payments are entered, depending on their billing procedures. In this chapter, you will be introduced to both methods of payment entry.

Patient payments—payments made to the practice directly by the patient or guarantor—are entered in the Transaction Entry dialog box. This method is convenient for entering a patient copayment made at the conclusion of an office visit.

Insurance payments—payments made to the practice on behalf of a patient by an insurance carrier—are entered in the Deposit List dialog box. The Deposit List feature is more efficient for entering large insurance payments that must be split up and applied to a number of different patients.

Patient Payments

Patient payments, like charges, are case-based. You must enter a patient's chart number and a case number before you can apply a payment to a patient's account. To record a patient payment, you must choose to enter a new transaction and then complete the required fields in the Payments, Adjustments, and Comments section of the Transaction Entry dialog box (see Figure 5-6 on page 86). You must enter a transaction date, payment/adjustment code, provider, and amount. You must also indicate who made the payment. The payment may be a copayment due at the time of the office visit or a check sent in the mail.

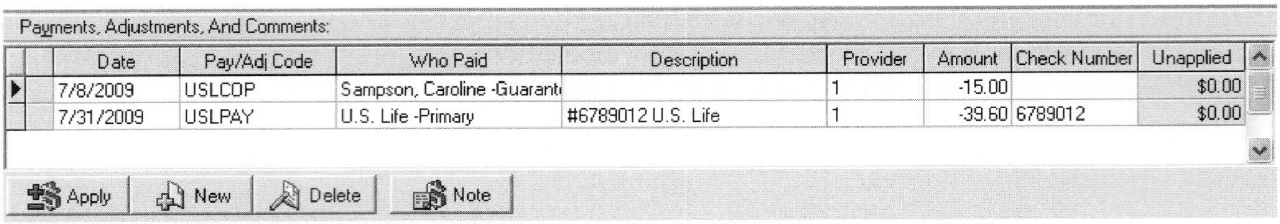

Payments, Adjustments, And Comments:

	Date	Pay/Adj Code	Who Paid	Description	Provider	Amount	Check Number	Unapplied
▶	7/8/2009	USLCOP	Sampson, Caroline -Guarant		1	-15.00		$0.00
	7/31/2009	USLPAY	U.S. Life -Primary	#6789012 U.S. Life	1	-39.60	6789012	$0.00

Apply   New   Delete   Note

Figure 5-6   Payments, Adjustments, and Comments Section of the Transaction Entry Dialog Box

One of the final steps in recording a payment is to apply the payment amount to one or more procedure charges. A typical charge could include two procedures ($60 and $25, for example). If a patient sent a check for $85, you must apply $60 to the first procedure and the remainder ($25) to the other procedure.

Printing a Walkout Receipt

After you complete a patient payment transaction, the NDCMedisoft™ program makes it easy to print a receipt for a patient. Just click the Print Receipt button to print a detailed receipt similar to the one shown in Figure 5-7. The patient information (name, diagnosis, charges, and amounts) pertaining to the case appears on the printout.

Computer Practice 5-5: *Recording a Charge and Copayment from a Patient (Hiro Tanaka)*

Review the encounter form for Hiro Tanaka shown in Source Document 14. At the time of the office visit, Tanaka's father paid the $10 copayment with check number 3022. Follow these steps to record the charge and payment for this patient, and then print a walkout receipt.

1. Verify that the NDCMedisoft™ Program Date is set to September 4, 2009.

2. Select the Enter Transactions option from the Activities menu, or use the toolbar to select this option.

3. Select Hiro Tanaka's chart number.

4. Since there is only one case for this patient, the case number automatically appears when you enter the chart number. If there were more than one case, you would have to select the appropriate case to see the corresponding charges. The program defaults to the most recent case.

5. Click the New button in the Charges area of the dialog box, and enter the procedure charge from the encounter form. You will also need to enter a charge for the insurance copayment—in this case, the code for the copayment charge is TRICOC—Tricare Copayment Charge. Click the New button again, and enter the copayment charge.

Family Care Center
285 Stephenson Boulevard
Stephenson, OH 60089
(614)555-0100

Patient:	Hal Sampson 3 Broadbrook Lane Stephenson, OH 60089
Chart #:	SAMHA000
Case #:	15

Instructions:
Complete the patient information portion of your insurance claim form. Attach this bill, signed and dated, and all other bills pertaining to the claim. If you have a deductible policy, hold your claim forms until you have met your deductible. Mail directly to your insurance carrier.

Date	Description	Procedure	Modify	Dx 1	Dx 2	Dx 3	Dx 4	Units	Charge
7/8/2009	OF--Established patient, low	99212		401.9				1	39.60
7/8/2009	USLife Copayment Charge	USLCOC		401.9				1	15.00
7/8/2009	USLife Patient Copayment	USLCOP						1	-15.00

Provider Information

Provider Name:	Katherine Yan M.D.
License:	84021
Commercial PIN:	60-3872-8
SSN or EIN:	810-99-1110

Total Charges:	$ 54.60
Total Payments:	-$ 15.00
Total Adjustments:	$ 0.00
Total Due This Visit:	**$ 39.60**
Total Account Balance:	$ 0.00

Assign and Release: I hereby authorize payment of medical benefits to this physician for the services described above. I also authorize the release of any information necessary to process this claim.

Patient Signature: _____ Date: _____

Figure 5-7 *Sample Walkout Receipt*

6. Now click the New button in the Payments, Adjustments, and Comments section to enter the payment transaction.

7. Select TRICOP—Tricare Patient Copayment—in the Pay/Adj Code box, and press Tab. Notice that the program automatically completes the Who Paid, Provider, and the Amount fields for you.

8. Record the check number in the Check Number field.

9. Click the Apply button to display the Apply Payment to Charges window, so that you can apply the $10.00 payment to the appropriate procedure charges.

10. Enter the payment amount in the This Payment field shown in the Apply Payment to Charges window for the 9/4/09 TRICARE copayment charge of $10.00. Click the Close button to close the Apply Payment to Charges window after you record the payment.

11. Click the Save Transactions button to save the data that you entered.

12. Review the information in the updated Transaction Entry window. If there are any errors, highlight the transaction, and then edit the entry. Notice that the payment is now shown in the lower half of the window. The payment appears as a negative amount (−10.00).

13. Now print a walkout receipt by clicking the Print Receipt button. In the box that appears, accept the default selection—Walkout Receipt (All Transactions). Then click the OK button.

14. In the Print Report Where? dialog box, accept the default selection to preview the report on the screen. Then click the Start button.

15. Accept the default date entries of 9/4/2009 in the Data Selection Questions box, and press OK.

16. Review the walkout receipt that appears on your screen. It should list the charge and payment transactions for September 4, 2009. When you are finished, close the Preview Report window.

17. Close the Transaction Entry dialog box.

Computer Practice 5-6: *Recording a Charge and Copayment, Creating a New Case, and Printing a Walkout Receipt (Elizabeth Jones)*

Review the encounter form for Elizabeth Jones (Source Document 15). After her office visit, Jones paid the $15 copayment with check number 609. Follow these steps to record the charge and payment and print a walkout receipt.

1. Verify that the NDCMedisoft™ Program Date is set to September 4, 2009.

2. Select the Enter Transactions option from the Activities menu, or use the toolbar to select this option.

3. Select Elizabeth Jones's chart number.

4. A case number appears, but today's visit is for another complaint. You could begin a new case by clicking in the Case field and pressing F8. However, there is a faster way to create a new case for an existing patient. Click Patients/Guarantors and Cases on the Lists menu.

5. Search for Jones in the list of patients. Then click the Case button.

6. Click the Copy Case button at the bottom of the dialog box. A new case appears, complete with all the information from the existing case. There is no need to reenter all the insurance information: it is entered for you. The only fields you need to change in this case are the Description field and the Diagnosis field. Enter the case description (use the diagnosis as the description), and enter the diagnosis in the Diagnosis tab.

7. Save the newly created case, and close the Patient List window. You are returned to the Transaction Entry window, with the new case active. Note: If the new case is not yet displayed, click the Update All button at the bottom of the Transaction Entry dialog box. Click Yes to re-save all the transactions if necessary. Then select the new case from the drop-down list in the Case field.

8. Click the New button in the Charges area, and enter the charge from the encounter form. Since a copayment is required by the patient's insurance company, you also need to enter a copayment charge. For this case, the code is USLCOC—U.S. Life Copayment Charge. Click the New button again, and enter the copayment charge.

9. Click the New button in the Payments, Adjustments, and Comments section. Select USLCOP—U.S. Life Patient Copayment—in the Pay/Adj Code box, and then press Tab.

10. Record the check number in the Check Number field.

11. Click the Apply button so that you can apply the $15.00 payment to the appropriate procedure charges.

12. Enter the payment amount in the This Payment field shown in the Apply Payment to Charges window. Apply the payment to the copayment charge for 9/4/09.

13. Click the Close button to close the Apply Payment to Charges window after you record the payment. Then save the transactions.

14. Review the latest information in the Transaction Entry window. If there are any errors, highlight the transaction, and then edit the entry. Notice that the payment is now shown in the lower half of the window. The payment appears as a negative amount (−15.00).

15. Using the steps you practiced in the previous exercise, preview a walkout receipt on your screen. It should list the charge and payment transactions for September 4, 2009. When you are finished, close the Preview Report window.

Computer Practice 5-7: *Using MultiLink Codes and Entering Modifiers (Sarina Bell)*

Review the encounter form for Sarina Bell (Source Document 16). You will use a single MultiLink code to record the procedures. You will also enter a modifier for one of the procedure codes. Bell's father, Herbert, paid the $15 copayment with check number 309. Follow these steps to record the charge and payment, and then print a walkout receipt.

1. Verify that the NDCMedisoft™ Program Date is set to September 4, 2009.

2. Open the Transaction Entry dialog box, if it is not already open.

3. Select Sarina Bell.

4. Create a new case. Complete the Personal, Account, Diagnosis, and Policy 1 tabs. Since Sarina's father, Herbert, is the guarantor, you can find the account and insurance information by looking at one of his cases.

5. Save the newly created case, and close the Patient List window if it is open. You are returned to the Transaction Entry window, with the new case active.

6. Click the MultiLink button. In the MultiLink Code box, choose STREP. Confirm that the Transaction Date entry is 9/4/2009 (if it is not, change the date to 9/4/2009). Then click the Create Transactions button. Notice that the program automatically entered all three codes for the office visit—99212, 87430, and 85025.

7. Now enter *90* in the first modifier (M1) box for procedure code 85025 (CBC w/diff).

8. Enter the $15.00 copayment charge for U.S. Life.

9. Click the New button in the Payments, Adjustments, and Comments area to enter the $15.00 payment. Then apply the payment to the appropriate charge.

10. Save the transactions, and print a walkout receipt.

11. Close the Transaction Entry dialog box.

Computer Practice 5-8: *Recording a Payment Received in the Mail (Caroline Mitchell)*

Family Care Center received check number 3024 in the amount of $60 from Caroline Mitchell for her June 15, 2009, office visit. Since she has not met her deductible, her insurance carrier, Blue Cross/Blue Shield, did not pay the claim. Enter the payment in the Transaction Entry tab.

1. Verify that the NDCMedisoft™ Program Date is set to September 4, 2009.

2. Open the Transaction Entry dialog box.

3. Select Mitchell's chart number.

4. Since there is only one case, you do not have to select the appropriate case to see the corresponding charges.

5. Enter the payment, using code 02—Patient payment, check—and apply it to the June 15, 2009, charge.

6. Save your work.

7. Preview a walkout receipt.

8. Close the Preview window.

9. Close the Transaction Entry dialog box.

Insurance Payments

Information about payments from insurance carriers is mailed or electronically transmitted to a physician through an electronic remittance advice. A **remittance advice (RA)** lists patients, dates of service, charges, and the amount paid or denied by the insurance carrier. Most RAs also provide explanations of unpaid charges. Sometimes a paper check is attached to the RA; in other cases the payment is deposited directly in the practice's bank account. Payment information located on the RA is entered in the Deposit List dialog box (see Figure 5-8). This dialog box is opened by clicking Enter Deposits/Payments on the Activities menu.

The first thing you need to do when entering a deposit is to enter the date of the deposit in the Deposit Date field. Once the correct date has been entered, click the New button to enter specific information about the deposit in the Deposit dialog box (see Figure 5-9 on page 92). First, select the option in the Payor Type field to indicate whether the payment is a patient, insurance, or capitation payment. Then you need to record the payment method, the check number, a description, the amount of the payment, and the insurance carrier that made the payment. When the insurance carrier field is completed, NDCMedisoft™ automatically

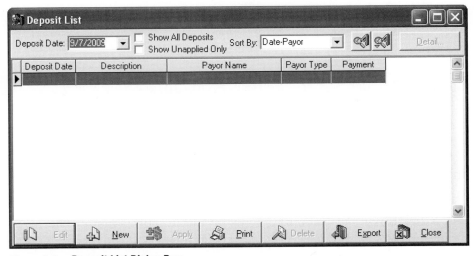

Figure 5-8 *Deposit List Dialog Box*

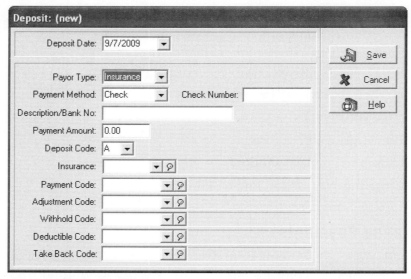

Figure 5-9 **Deposit Dialog Box**

completes the code fields at the bottom of the dialog box. After you have completed the entries and checked your work for accuracy, click the Save button. Your entry now appears in the Deposit List dialog box.

Insurance payments must be applied to specific patients, cases, dates, and procedures. To do this, click the Apply button in the Deposit List dialog box. Notice that the amount of the payment appears in the upper right corner under the heading Unapplied. As you apply payments, this amount will decrease until it reaches zero. To begin applying the payment, select a patient's chart number in the For field. The program then lists that patient's unpaid charges. Using information on the RA, enter the appropriate payment amounts in the Payment column for each procedure charge, and press the Tab key. When you are finished entering payments for that patient, save your work by clicking the Save Payments/Adjustments button.

If the payment is for more than one patient, you can continue applying the payment by selecting the next patient in the For field. Remember to click the Save Payments/Adjustments button each time you finish working with a specific patient. You should apply payments until the unapplied amount for the deposit is zero.

Computer Practice 5-9: *Recording Payments from an Insurance Carrier*

Family Care Center received an RA from Blue Cross/Blue Shield for several patients. Enter the deposit, and apply the payments using the information from Source Document 17.

1. Change the NDCMedisoft™ Program Date to September 7, 2009.

2. Click Enter Deposits/Payments on the Activities menu. The Deposit List dialog box is displayed. Verify that the correct date appears in the Deposit Date field.

3. Click the New button. A Confirm dialog box appears, indicating that you have entered a future date and asking whether you want to change the date. Click the No button. Then click the New button again. The Deposit (new) dialog box is displayed.

4. Confirm that the entry in the Deposit Date box is 9/7/2009.

5. Since this is a payment from an insurance carrier, make sure that the selection in the Payor Type box is Insurance.

6. Enter Electronic in the Payment Method box.

7. Enter *36094251* in the EFT Tracer box.

8. The Description/Bank No. field can be left blank.

9. Key *575.20* in the Payment Amount box.

10. Accept the default entry (A) in the Deposit Code box.

11. Select 4—Blue Cross/Blue Shield—from the Insurance drop-down list. When an insurance carrier is selected in the Insurance box, NDCMedisoft™ automatically enters codes in the remaining fields.

12. Click the Save button to save the entry. The Deposit dialog box closes.

13. The Deposit List box reappears. The insurance payment appears in the list of deposits. Now the payment must be applied to the specific procedure charges to which it is related.

14. With the Blue Cross/Blue Shield payment entry highlighted, click the Apply button. The Apply Payment/Adjustments to Charges dialog box appears (see Figure 5-10).

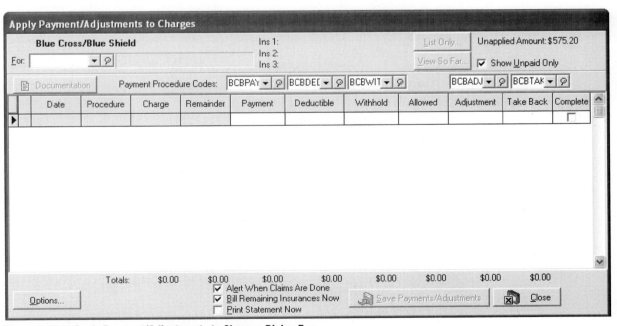

Figure 5-10 *Apply Payment/Adjustments to Charges Dialog Box*

15. Key *F* in the For box, and press Enter to select Stanley Feldman, since he is listed on the RA. All the charge entries for Feldman that have not been paid in full are listed.

16. Since this payment is for the 93015 procedure completed on 7/28/09, that is the line in which the payment will be applied. Notice that the cursor is flashing in the Payment box.

17. Key *260* in the Payment box, and press Enter. NDCMedisoft™ automatically places a minus sign before the amount. Continue to press Enter until the amount listed in the Remainder column adjusts. Notice that once the payment was applied, the Complete box to the right of the dialog box was checked.

18. Click the Save Payments/Adjustments button to save your entry. An Information box appears, stating that the claim has been marked done for the primary insurance carrier. Click the OK button. The dialog box is cleared of the current transactions and is ready for a new transaction. Notice that the Unapplied Amount in the upper right corner of the dialog box has been reduced to $315.20.

19. Select Marion Johnson from the For list, and apply the Blue Cross/Blue Shield payments to her July 15, 2009, and August 18, 2009, charges. When you are done, save your work. Notice that the Unapplied Amount is now $70.40.

20. Select James Smith, and apply the payments to his July 8, 2009, and August 17, 2009, charges. Before you click the button to save your work, notice that the Unapplied Amount is now 0.00. Then save your work.

21. Click the Close button to exit the Apply Payment/Adjustments to Charges dialog box.

Adjustments

Occasionally, it may be necessary to make an adjustment to a patient's account. For example, an insurance company may pay for a lesser procedure than the one submitted by the practice. Adjustments are noted on RAs received from the carriers.

Computer Practice 5-10: *Entering an Adjustment*

Use the information on Source Document 18 to enter an adjustment for Ellen Barmenstein's September 4, 2009, office visit.

1. Open the Deposit List dialog box, if it is not already open.

2. Verify that the Deposit Date is September 7, 2009.

3. Click the New button.

4. Enter the information about the payment in the Deposit dialog box, and click the Save button.

5. With the payment highlighted in the Deposit List window, click the Apply button.

6. Select Barmenstein's chart number.

7. Enter the payment for the charge on August 28, 2009.

8. Enter the zero payment for the first charge listed (99211) for September 4, 2009, and then press Enter.

9. Apply the deposit to the other two charges.

10. Save the entry, and close the Apply Payment/Adjustments to Charges dialog box.

11. Close the Deposit List dialog box.

✓CHECKPOINT

4. Which application menu option do you use to enter a patient payment?

5. Which option do you use to assign a patient payment to a particular procedure charge?

6. Which application menu option do you use to enter an insurance carrier payment?

Computer Practice 5-11: Exiting the Program and Making a Backup Copy

Practice quitting the software and making a backup copy of your work by following these steps:

1. Choose Exit from the File menu, or use the toolbar to select this option.

2. Insert your working copy of the Student Data Disk in Drive A:.

3. Click the Back Up Data Now button.

4. In the Destination File Path and Name box, enter *A:\PBChap5.mbk.*

5. Click the Start Backup button. When the Backup Complete box appears, click OK. The NDCMedisoft™ program shuts down.

6. Remove the floppy disk from Drive A:.

7. Store your disk in a safe place.

CHAPTER 5 Review

DEFINE THE TERMS

Write a definition for each term: (Obj. 5-1)

1. Charge

   _____

2. Outpatient

   _____

3. MultiLink code

   _____

4. Insurance payments

   _____

5. Modifiers

   _____

6. Default

   _____

7. Patient payments

   _____

8. Inpatient

   _____

9. Adjustment

   _____

10. Remittance advice (RA)

    _____

11. What are the steps required to record a procedure charge? (Objs. 5-2, 5-3)

   _____

   _____

   _____

12. How do you record a payment from a patient? Why is it necessary to apply the payment to specific charges? (Obj. 5-4)

   _____

   _____

   _____

13. To enter a procedure charge, do you have to identify the patient's chart number and case number? What steps are required if a case has not been set up? (Obj. 5-3)

   _____

   _____

14. What information is printed on a walkout receipt? (Obj. 5-5)

   _____

   _____

15. Where is an adjustment entered? (Obj. 5-6)

   _____

CRITICAL ANALYSIS EXERCISE

16. Why does the NDCMedisoft™ program organize transactions based on patient cases? (Objs. 5-3, 5-4)

   _____

   _____

   _____

   _____

Processing Claims and Creating Statements

WHAT YOU NEED TO KNOW

To complete this chapter, you need to know how to:

- Enter information in NDCMedisoft™.
- Navigate the NDCMedisoft™ software.
- Search for information in an NDCMedisoft™ database.
- Enter patient and case information.
- Record procedure charges and payments.

WHAT YOU WILL LEARN

When you finish this chapter, you will be able to:

1. Define the terms introduced in this chapter.
2. Describe the claim management process.
3. Create claims.
4. Edit claim information.
5. Describe the steps required to transmit electronic claims.
6. Explain how to mark and delete claims.
7. Describe the different types of patient statements.
8. Create and print patient statements.

KEY TERMS

Claim status The current disposition of a medical claim.

Clearinghouse A service bureau that collects electronic claims from many different medical practices and forwards them to the appropriate insurance carriers.

Cycle billing A patient billing system in which patients are divided into groups and statement printing and mailing is staggered throughout the month.

EDI receiver An insurance company or clearinghouse set up to electronically receive and process insurance claims submitted by the medical practice.

Once-a-month billing A patient billing system in which all statements are printed and mailed once a month, all at the same time.

Patient statement A list of the amount of money a patient owes, organized by the amount of time the money has been owed, the procedures performed, and the dates the procedures were performed.

Remainder statements Statements that list only those charges that are not paid in full after all insurance carrier payments have been received.

Standard statements Statements that show all charges regardless of whether the insurance has paid on the transactions.

Claim Management

Claim management is an important activity in the patient billing process. Processing claims involves creating claims, editing them (if necessary), and sending them to various insurance companies for payment. Claims can be sent electronically or on paper, and the NDCMedisoft™ program can accommodate either method. In this tutorial, however, you will focus on electronic claims.

Depending on the medical practice, a billing assistant may process claims on a daily or weekly basis. The Family Care Center processes claims on a daily basis. As you work through this chapter, you will learn how to process claims. In NDCMedisoft™, claims are processed using the Claim Management option in the Activities menu. When you select this option, NDCMedisoft™ displays the Claim Management window as shown in Figure 6-1. As you can see, this window includes options to edit, create, print/send, reprint, and delete claims. You will learn how to use each of these options in the following sections.

As you use the NDCMedisoft™ program, the list of claims in the Claim Management window will continue to expand. Each day you will add new claims to the list of those that have already been sent. Some claims may be marked as challenged or rejected, while others may be held for processing. From time to time, you can remove or delete claims after you no longer need the information.

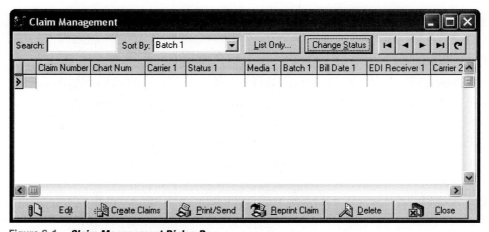

Figure 6-1 *Claim Management Dialog Box*

Creating Claims

After you enter procedure charges, the next step is to create the insurance claims. The NDCMedisoft™ program simplifies this task by automating many aspects of the claim creation process. Using the Claim Management capabilities, you can create claims for all procedure charges, or you can direct the program to create claims that match certain criteria. For example, you can create claims for all charges entered on a certain date or for a specific insurance carrier. These options and others are available in the Create Claims window (see Figure 6-2).

After you decide which claims you want to create, the NDCMedisoft™ program generates the claims based on the procedure charges, insurance policy data, and other information you entered for each case. The program looks at each charge to determine whether it should create a claim. If a patient is not covered by a health insurance policy or you have not entered the policy information, the program will not create a claim for that procedure charge. If a claim has already been created for a procedure charge, a new claim is not created.

After the program determines which claims to generate, it automatically creates them, assigns each a claim number, and displays them in the Claim Management window (see Figure 6-3 on page 102). As shown in the figure, the status of the new claims is Ready to Send, and the billing method or media is set to EDI, for electronic data interchange, meaning the claims will be sent electronically. **Claim status** refers to the current disposition of a claim. With NDCMedisoft™, you can change the claim status to any of the following: Hold, Ready to Send, Sent, Rejected, Challenge, Alert, Done, and Pending.

The Claim Management window also includes a column to show the EDI receiver. An **EDI receiver** is an insurance company or clearinghouse set up to electronically receive and process insurance claims submitted by the medical practice. A **clearinghouse** is a service bureau that collects electronic insurance claims from many different medical practices and forwards them to the appropriate insurance carriers.

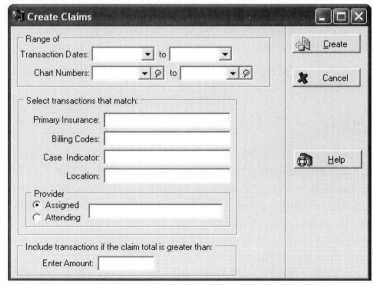

Figure 6-2 *Create Claims Dialog Box*

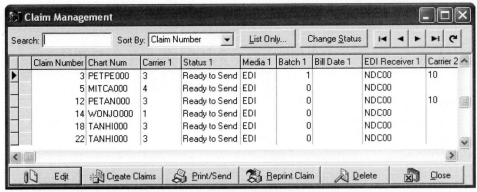

Figure 6-3   *Claims Displayed in the Claim Management Dialog Box*

Computer Practice 6-1: *Creating Claims*

The Family Care Center processes new claims every day. Follow the steps provided below to create the insurance claims for the transactions that you entered on September 4, 2009.

1. Start the NDCMedisoft™ program.

2. Set the program date to September 4, 2009.

3. Restore the backup file that you created at the end of Chapter 5.

4. Pull down the Activities menu, and choose the Claim Management option to display the Claim Management window.

5. Click the Create Claims button to display the window that lets you specify which claims to create.

6. Enter *9/4/2009* in both of the Transaction Dates fields so that the program will create the claims for that date only. Note: The confirm dialog box will remind you that you have entered a future date. In answer to the question about whether you want to change the date, click the No button.

7. Click the Create button in the Create Claims window to generate the claims for the transactions recorded on September 4, 2009.

8. Review the claims that are listed in the Claim Management window.

Editing Claims

You can edit any of the claims that appear in the Claim Management window. Although the claim information generated by the NDCMedisoft™ program is usually correct, you may have a reason to change some of this information. For example, you could change the status for a specific claim from Sent to Rejected if a claim has been rejected by an insurance carrier. Or you could select a different insurance carrier if this information was incorrectly recorded in a patient's case.

To edit a claim, simply highlight the claim and click the Edit button. When you choose to edit a claim, the NDCMedisoft™ program displays the

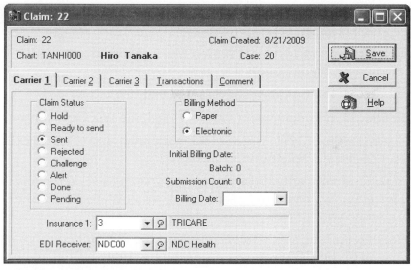

Figure 6-4   *Claim Dialog Box*

Claim window as shown in Figure 6-4. As you can see, you can change the claim status, billing method, billing date, insurance carrier, or EDI receiver. Using this option, you can also view the transactions associated with a claim or attach a comment.

Computer Practice 6-2: *Editing Claims*

Follow the steps listed here to learn how you can review and edit the information stored for a claim:

1. Verify that the program date is set to 9/4/09.

2. Select (highlight) any one of the claims shown in the Claim Management window.

3. Click the Edit button to view and update the claim you chose.

4. Review the information in the Carrier 1, Carrier 2, and Carrier 3 folders by clicking the appropriate tab, but do not change any of the data.

5. Click the Transactions tab to review the transaction data.

6. Close the Cancel button to close the Claim dialog box.

Proofing Claims Using the List Only Option

As the list of previously sent claims grows, it can be difficult to verify the new claims to be sent. The List Only feature is useful in proofing new claims. You can use this option to list only those claims created on a certain date or to be sent to a specific carrier. After you use this option, you should always select it again and reset the criteria to the defaults so that all of the claims appear in the Claim Management window.

Computer Practice 6-3: *Reviewing Insurance Claims*

Learn how to use the List Only option to review insurance claims before you send them. Follow the steps provided here:

1. Verify that the program date is set to 9/4/09.

2. In the Claim Management window, click the List Only button.

3. Select 4—Blue Cross/Blue Shield in the Insurance Carrier field, and click the Apply button.

4. You should see only those claims that match the criteria you set. However, you could have selected several different criteria to fine-tune your search.

5. Before you continue, you need to reset the List Only options so that all of the claims appear. Click the List Only button again to display the List Only Claims That Match window. Click the Defaults button to reset all of the options, and then click the Apply button.

6. Verify that all of the claims appear in the list.

7. Close the Claim Management dialog box.

Transmitting Electronic Claims

In an actual office setting, the claims that you just created would have been sent to the clearinghouse or insurance carrier. Because schools are not set up to transmit electronic claims, Exercise 6-3 above ends without actually transmitting claims. The steps below describe the process of actually transmitting electronic claims.

Computer Practice 6-4: *Prepare to Transmit Electronic Claims*

Practice the steps that you would follow to transmit electronic claims in NDCMedisoft™.

1. Click Claim Management on the Activities menu.

2. Click the Print/Send button.

3. In the Print/Send Claims dialog box, click the Electronic button to change the billing method to electronic, if it is not already selected. Set the Electronic Claim Receiver box to NDC, which stands for National Data Corporation, if it is not already set.

4. Click the OK button. The Send Electronic Claims dialog box is displayed, with National Data Corporation displayed as the receiver.

5. Click the Send Claims Now button.

6. The Data Selection Questions dialog box appears. The various range boxes provide options for filtering the claims. For now, leave the range boxes as they are, and click the OK button.

7. An Information dialog box appears, asking whether to display a Verification report. After clicking Yes, the Preview Report window appears with a copy of an EMC Verification report displayed. The report displays the details of each claim in the batch. Click the Close button when finished viewing the report. The Preview Report window closes, and an Information dialog box appears, asking you if you want to continue with the transmission.

8. If you were in a medical office, you would click the Yes button, and the claim would be sent via cable lines, telephone lines, or satellite from your computer to a computer at the clearinghouse. However, because you are in a school setting and are not set up to submit electronic claims at this time, click the No button.

9. Click the Close button to close the Claim Management dialog box and return to the main NDCMedisoft™ window.

Sending Electronic Claim Attachments

When sending a claim electronically, an attachment that needs to accompany the claim, such as radiology films, must be referred to in the claim. In NDCMedisoft™, the EDI Report area within the Diagnosis tab of the Case dialog box is used to indicate to the payer when an attachment will accompany the claim and how the attachment will be transmitted.

Printing Insurance Claim Forms

Occasionally it is necessary to print and mail some claims rather than transmit them electronically. To print a claim, you first must determine whether the claim is listed as electronic or paper in the Claim Management dialog box. If it is listed as EDI, you will need to edit the claim and change the billing method to paper in order to print the claim. Then you will be able to print it using the same Print/Send button that you would use to send electronic claims.

You must also select the appropriate paper claim report format. For our purposes, you should always use the HCFA-1500 (Primary) report. When you preview a report or print the final claim forms, the data may not seem to be formatted properly. Remember that a medical office must print the claims on forms and send the completed forms to the respective insurance carriers. The location of the data corresponds to the required fields on the form.

Once a claim has been printed (or transmitted electronically), the NDCMedisoft™ program changes the claim status from Ready to Send to Sent.

Computer Practice 6-5: *Printing Insurance Claims*

Follow the instructions provided below to print insurance claim forms. Since all insurance claims in this text/workbook are set up to be transmitted electronically, you will need to change the billing method to Paper for this exercise.

1. Verify that the program date is set to 9/4/09.

2. Open the Claim Management window, select the claim for Peter Peterson (PETPE000), and click the Edit button.

3. Change the Billing Method from Electronic to Paper, and click the Save button.

4. Click the Print/Send button. Make sure that you have selected the option to print claims using the paper billing method. Click the OK button to continue.

5. In the Open Report window, choose the HCFA-1500 (Primary) report, and click the OK button.

6. Choose to preview the reports on the screen.

7. Accept the default settings in the Data Selection Questions window.

8. Review the claim.

9. Print the claim unless you are instructed otherwise. Note: If you do not actually print the claim, the Claim Status will not change from Ready to Send to Sent.

10. Close the report window.

11. Review the status of the claims.

12. Close the Claim Management window.

Marking Accepted Claims

If you need to manually mark a claim, you can edit it and change the status by choosing the appropriate option. You may, for example, need to change the status of a claim from Rejected to Hold.

When you print claims, the software automatically changes the status to Sent. If you send claims electronically and a link is established to receive an audit/edit report, the software can also be set up to automatically mark whether a claim was accepted, challenged, or rejected. Since it is not possible to actually send electronic claims during these exercises, the claim status needs to be manually updated from Ready to Send to Sent.

Computer Practice 6-6: *Changing the Status of Claims*

Change the claim status for the claims created on September 4, 2009 from Ready to Send to Sent.

1. Open the Claim Management dialog box.

2. In the Claim Management dialog box, click the Change Status button. The Change Claim Status/Billing Method dialog box appears.

3. Click the Batch radio button, and enter *0* in the box to the right.

4. Select Ready to Send in the Status From column.

5. Select Sent in the Status To column.

6. Click the OK button. The dialog box closes, and the Claim Management dialog box reappears with the Status 1 column displaying Sent.

7. Close the Claim Management dialog box.

Deleting Claims

Using the Claim Management functions, you can delete claims that are no longer needed so that the list of claims is more manageable. Although many medical practices leave sent claims active for quite some time, you can remove the old claims that have been paid by the insurance carriers. For our purposes, you should not need to delete any claims that you create.

What if you accidentally create claims that should not be included in the list? Rather than deleting the claims, you could mark them as Hold. This method is preferable to deleting the claims.

✓CHECKPOINT

1. Which menu contains the Claim Management feature?

2. Using the Claim Management window, which button lets you create new claims?

3. What status is assigned to a claim before it is printed or sent?

4. After claims are transmitted, what status does the program use to mark those claims?

Creating Patient Statements

A **patient statement** lists the amount of money a patient owes, organized by the amount of time the money has been owed, the procedures performed, and the dates the procedures were performed (see Figure 6-5 on page 108 for a sample statement). In earlier versions of NDCMedisoft™, statements were created from the Reports menu. Beginning with Version 9, statements are created using the new Statement Management feature, which is listed on the Activities menu.

Just as Claim Management provides a range of options for billing insurance carriers, Statement Management offers multiple choices for billing patients. Within the Statement Management area of NDCMedisoft™, statements are created and printed.

Statement Management Dialog Box

The Statement Management dialog box, as illustrated in Figure 6-6 on page 109, is displayed by clicking Statement Management on the Activities menu or by clicking the shortcut button on the toolbar.

Creating Patient Statements

After you enter, create, transmit, and process insurance claims, it is time to create patient statements. Statements are created in the Create Statements dialog box (see Figure 6-7 on page 109).

Family Care Center

285 Stephenson Boulevard

Stephenson, OH 60089

(614)555-0100

Statement Date	Chart Number	Page
09/07/2009	BAREL000	1

Ellen Barmenstein

1774 Grand Street

Stephenson, OH 60089

Make Checks Payable To:
Family Care Center
285 Stephenson Boulevard
Stephenson, OH 60089
(614)555-0100

Date of Last Payment: 9/7/2009	Amount: -9.60	Previous Balance:	0.00

Patient:	Ellen Barmenstein		Chart Number: BAREL000		Case:	Office Visit		
Dates	Procedure	Charge	Paid by Primary		Paid By Guarantor	Adjustments	Remainder
08/28/09	99212	44.00	-35.20			0.00	8.80

Patient:	Ellen Barmenstein		Chart Number: BAREL000		Case:	Flu immunization		
Dates	Procedure	Charge	Paid by Primary		Paid By Guarantor	Adjustments	Remainder
09/04/09	99211	30.00	0.00			0.00	30.00
09/04/09	90471	10.00	-8.00			0.00	2.00
09/04/09	90658	12.00	-9.60			0.00	2.40

Amount Due
43.20

Figure 6-5   *Sample Patient Statement*

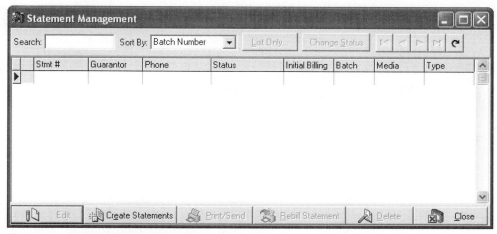

Figure 6-6   Statement Management Dialog Box

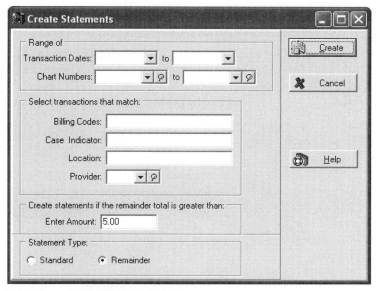

Figure 6-7   Create Statements Dialog Box

Using the Statement Management feature, you can create statements for all transactions, or you can create only those statements that match certain criteria. In the Create Statements dialog box, statements can be filtered by transaction dates, chart numbers, billing codes, case indicator, location, and provider.

There is also an option to limit the creation of statements to accounts that have a balance of a certain dollar amount or more. For example, a practice may have a policy that statements are not mailed to patients whose accounts have a balance below $5.

In addition, the type of statement must be specified. NDCMedisoft™ offers two options: standard and remainder. **Standard statements** show all available charges regardless of whether the insurance has paid on the transactions. **Remainder statements** list only those charges that are not paid in full after all insurance carrier payments have been received. Once a statement type is selected, the setting remains in effect until the other type of statement is selected.

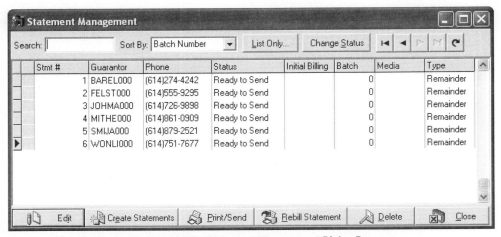

Figure 6-8 *Statements Displayed in the Statement Management Dialog Box*

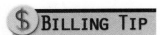
After all selections are complete in the Create Statements dialog box, clicking the Create button instructs the program to generate statements. The NDCMedisoft™ application looks at each charge to determine whether it has been paid in full or a balance remains. After the program determines which statements to generate, it automatically creates the statements, assigns numbers, and displays a list of the statements in the Statement Management window (see Figure 6-8). As shown in the figure, the claim status of the new statements is Ready to Send, and the Type is Remainder.

Computer Practice 6-7: *Creating Statements*

Create remainder statements for all patients with outstanding balances of $5 or more.

1. Select Statement Management on the Activities menu.

2. Click the Create Statements button.

3. Verify that 5.00 is displayed in the Create Statements if the Remainder Total Is Greater Than field. Make sure that the Remainder radio button is selected in the Statement Type box. Leave all other boxes as they are.

4. Click the Create button. A message is displayed indicating the number of statements that were created.

5. Click the OK button.

6. The Statement Management dialog box displays the list of statements that were created.

Printing Statements

Once statements have been created, the next step is to print them on a printer or send them electronically. When the Print/Send button is clicked, the Print/Send Statements dialog box is displayed (see Figure 6-9). This box lists options for choosing the type of statement that will be created—

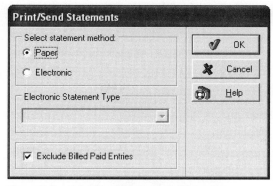

Figure 6-9 *Print/Send Statements Dialog Box*

Paper or Electronic. Paper statements are printed and mailed by the practice. Electronic statements are sent electronically to a processing center where statements are printed and mailed.

Once these selections are made, the OK button is clicked, and the Open Report dialog box appears. The report selected in this dialog box must match the type of statement selected in the Statement Type field of the Create Statements dialog box—either Standard or Remainder. If Remainder was checked, statements will print only if one of the three Remainder Statement report formats is selected in the Open Report window. The same is true for Standard Statements.

After the report format is selected, click the OK button to display the Print Report Where? dialog box, which asks whether to preview the report on screen, send the report directly to the printer, or export the report to a file.

Once the Start button is clicked, the Data Selection Questions dialog box appears. The fields in the Data Selection Questions dialog box are used to filter statement selections. For example, to print statements for a certain group of patients, entries are made in the Chart Number Range field. Many practices use cycle billing rather than once-a-month billing. In **once-a-month billing,** all statements are printed and mailed at once. In a **cycle billing** system, patients are divided into groups, and statement printing and mailing is staggered throughout the month. For example, statements for guarantors whose last names begin with the letters *A* to *F* are mailed on the first of the month; those with last names that begin with *G* to *L* are mailed on the eighth of the month; and so on.

In addition to the Chart Number Range filter, a number of additional filters are available, including a filter for selecting dates, insurance carriers, account balances, and other options. Once all selections are complete, clicking the OK button sends the statements to a printer, to an electronic statement processor, or to a file.

Computer Practice 6-8: *Printing Patient Statements*

1. Click the Print/Send button in the Statement Management dialog box.

2. Verify that the statement method button for paper is selected. Click the OK button.

3. Click Remainder Statement—All Payments, and then click the OK button.

4. Choose to preview the report on the screen.

5. Enter *BAREL000* in both of the Chart Number Range fields to print a patient statement for Ellen Barmenstein only.

6. Enter *8/1/2009* and *9/7/2009* in the Date From Range boxes. Then click the OK button.

7. Review the patient statement.

8. Print the report, but make sure that this report includes only one statement.

9. Notice that the status of the statement is now Sent.

10. Close the Statement Management dialog box.

✓CHECKPOINT

5. Which option from the Activities menu do you select to access the Statement Management functions?

6. If a patient has a zero balance, will NDCMedisoft™ create a statement for that patient?

7. Which type of statement lists all charges, regardless of whether a payment has been made?

8. After statements are printed, what status does the program assign to those statements?

Computer Practice 6-9: *Exiting the Program and Making a Backup Copy*

Practice quitting the software and making a backup copy of your work by following these steps:

1. Choose Exit from the File menu, or use the toolbar to select this option.

2. Insert your working copy of the Student Data Disk in Drive A:.

3. Click the Back Up Data Now button.

4. In the Destination File Path and Name box, enter *A:\PBChap6.mbk.*

5. Click the Start Backup button. When the Backup Complete box appears, click OK. The NDCMedisoft™ program shuts down.

6. Remove the floppy disk from Drive A:.

7. Store your disk in a safe place.

CHAPTER 6 Review

DEFINE THE TERMS

Write a definition for each term: (Obj. 6-1)

1. Claim status

   _____

2. Clearinghouse

   _____

3. Cycle billing

   _____

4. EDI receiver

   _____

5. Once-a-month billing

   _____

6. Patient statement

   _____

7. Remainder statements

   _____

8. Standard statements

   _____

CHECK YOUR UNDERSTANDING

9. What status does the program assign to new claims it creates? What other status options are used by the program? (Obj. 6-6)

   _____

   _____

10. What steps are required to transmit electronic claims that you already created? (Objs. 6-2, 6-5)

    _____

11. Can you edit claims after you create them? Why might you need to edit a claim? (Obj. 6-4)

_____

_____

12. When does the NDCMedisoft™ program automatically mark claims to indicate that they were sent? (Objs. 6-2, 6-4, 6-5, 6-6)

_____

_____

13. Why would you use the option to delete a claim? (Obj. 6-6)

_____

14. What type of statement would you choose if you wanted to bill a patient for the amount due after all payments were received from insurance carriers? (Obj. 6-7)

_____

15. What dialog box is used to filter statements before they are printed? (Obj. 6-8)

_____

CRITICAL ANALYSIS EXERCISES

16. List the steps to create and process claims. (Obj. 6-2)

_____

_____

_____

17. List the steps to create statements for all patients with account balances above $1. (Obj. 6-8)

_____

_____

_____

Producing Reports

WHAT YOU NEED TO KNOW

To complete this chapter, you need to know how to:

- Enter information in NDCMedisoft™.
- Navigate the NDCMedisoft™ software.
- Search for information in an NDCMedisoft™ database.
- Enter patient and case information.
- Record procedure charges and payments.

WHAT YOU WILL LEARN

When you finish this chapter, you will be able to:

1. Define the terms introduced in this chapter.
2. Describe the steps used to print a report.
3. Print Patient Day Sheet and Procedure Day Sheet reports.
4. Create two types of analysis reports.
5. Print a Patient Aging report.
6. Discuss the purpose of collection reports.
7. Print a Patient Ledger.
8. Print various list reports.
9. Describe how to create a custom report.

KEY TERMS

Aging The classification of accounts receivable by the length of time an account is past due.

Billing/Payment Status report A report that lists the status of all transactions, showing who has paid and who has not been billed.

Cash flow Movement of money into a practice from patients and out of a practice to suppliers and staff. Refers to actual cash as opposed to receivables and payables.

Insurance Aging report A report that shows an aging analysis of insurance accounts.

Insurance Collection reports Reports that are used to monitor outstanding claim balances of insurance carriers.

Patient Aging report A detailed report that shows an aging analysis of patient accounts.

Patient Collection report A report that is used to identify outstanding patient balances and monitor the collections process.

Patient Ledger report A report that lists the account activity for each patient for a specified time period and shows the current balance and any unpaid charges.

Payables Money owed by a practice, but not yet sent to suppliers.

Practice Analysis report Detailed report that shows the practice's revenue for a period of time.

Receivables Money owed to a medical practice, but not yet received from patients and insurance companies.

NDCMedisoft™ Reports

Reports provide a summary of the data stored in a database. An example is the report used by NDCMedisoft™ to track patient billing transactions. The reports produced by the NDCMedisoft™ program contain a variety of useful information about a medical practice and its patients.

The office manager, the providers, and you, as the billing assistant, may have different informational needs for the data provided on the various reports. For example, you might use the Patient Day Sheet to verify a bank deposit since this report shows the cash received during the day. Other reports may help the office manager track the medical practice's **cash flow**, or movement of money into and out of the practice.

Information regarding receivables and payables is used along with aging data to manage the financial aspects of a medical practice. **Receivables**, which represent money owed to a practice by its patients and insurance carriers, must be constantly tracked. Reports that show aging data classify receivables by the length of time an account is past due. An office manager could use these data to find out which patients or companies have accounts that are past due. **Payables**, or amounts due to suppliers, must be managed, too.

Some of the reports that you can print using the NDCMedisoft™ program are listed below. These reports are accessed via the Reports menu (see Figure 7-1).

Day Sheets

Day Sheet reports summarize activity during a specific period. Typically, these reports are printed at the end of each day. You can use them as a backup for the day's transactions, to verify the cash on hand with the receipts listed on the report, and to analyze the revenue for the day.

The Patient Day Sheet summarizes the procedures, charges, payments, and adjustments by patient. The Procedure Day Sheet provides similar information, but it is organized by procedure codes.

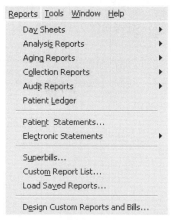

Figure 7-1   *NDCMedisoft™ Reports Menu*

Computer Practice 7-1: *Printing a Patient Day Sheet*

1. Start the NDCMedisoft™ program.

2. Set the program date to September 4, 2009.

3. Restore the backup file that you created at the end of Chapter 6.

4. Pull down the Reports menu, choose Day Sheets, and then choose the Patient Day Sheet option.

5. When the Print Report Where? dialog box appears, confirm that the Preview the Report on the Screen option is selected.

6. Click the Start button.

7. Delete the entries in the Date Created Range boxes (simply tab to the field and press the Delete key).

8. In the Date From Range fields, enter **9/4/2009** for the beginning and ending dates to print a Day Sheet for September 4, 2009, only (see Figure 7-2).

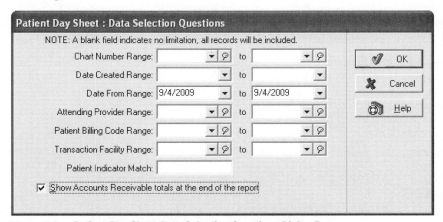

Figure 7-2   *Patient Day Sheet Data Selection Questions Dialog Box*

9. Click the box at the bottom of the window to show the accounts receivable totals at the end of the report. Then click the OK button.

Family Care Center

Patient Day Sheet
Ending 9/4/2009

Entry	Date	Document	POS	Description	Provider	Code	Modifier	Amount
BAREL000		**Ellen Barmenstein**						
205	9/4/2009	0909040000	11		1	99211		30.00
206	9/4/2009	0909040000	11		1	90471		10.00
207	9/4/2009	0909040000	11		1	90658		12.00
		Patient's Charges		Patient's Receipts		Adjustments		Patient Balance
		$52.00		$0.00		$0.00		$43.20
BELSA001		**Sarina Bell**						
214	9/4/2009	0909040000	11		1	99212		39.60
215	9/4/2009	0909040000	11		1	87430		28.80
216	9/4/2009	0909040000	11		1	85025	90	22.50
217	9/4/2009	0909040000	11		1	USLCOC		15.00
218	9/4/2009	0909040000	11		1	USLCOP		-15.00
		Patient's Charges		Patient's Receipts		Adjustments		Patient Balance
		$105.90		-$15.00		$0.00		$90.90
JONEL000		**Elizabeth Jones**						
211	9/4/2009	0909040000	11		1	99212		39.60
212	9/4/2009	0909040000	11		1	USLCOC		15.00
213	9/4/2009	0909040000	11		1	USLCOP		-15.00
		Patient's Charges		Patient's Receipts		Adjustments		Patient Balance
		$54.60		-$15.00		$0.00		$39.60
LOMCE000		**Cedera Lomos**						
198	9/4/2009	0909040000	11		1	99204		147.00
		Patient's Charges		Patient's Receipts		Adjustments		Patient Balance
		$147.00		$0.00		$0.00		$147.00
LOMLI000		**Lisa Lomos**						
201	9/4/2009	0909040000	11		1	90707		105.00
199	9/4/2009	0909040000	11		1	99383		140.00
200	9/4/2009	0909040000	11		1	90471		10.00
		Patient's Charges		Patient's Receipts		Adjustments		Patient Balance
		$255.00		$0.00		$0.00		$255.00
MITCA000		**Caroline Mitchell**						
219	9/4/2009	0909040000	11		1	02		-60.00
		Patient's Charges		Patient's Receipts		Adjustments		Patient Balance
		$0.00		-$60.00		$0.00		$0.00
PATLE000		**Leila Patterson**						
204	9/4/2009	0909040000	11		1	82465		21.00
203	9/4/2009	0909040000	11		1	99212		44.00
		Patient's Charges		Patient's Receipts		Adjustments		Patient Balance
		$65.00		$0.00		$0.00		$65.00
TANHI000		**Hiro Tanaka**						
208	9/4/2009	0909040000	11		1	99212		28.00
209	9/4/2009	0909040000	11		1	TRICOC		10.00

Figure 7-3 *Sample Preview of Patient Day Sheet Report*

10. After a few moments, the report should appear on your screen as shown in Figure 7-3. The buttons in the Preview Report window let you zoom the report, move from page to page, print the report, save it to disk, and close the report window.

11. Click the Zoom to Width of Page button (third button from the left) so that you can read the report information.

12. Scan the information shown on the report.

13. Click the Next Page (right arrow) button to view each of the report pages.

14. Click the Printer button to print the report.

15. Click the Close button to exit the Preview Report window.

Computer Practice 7-2: *Printing a Procedure Day Sheet*

1. Be sure the program date is set to 9/4/2009.

2. Select the option to print a Procedure Day Sheet.

3. Select the option to preview the report on your screen.

4. Tab to the entries in the Date Created Range boxes and delete both entries.

5. Enter *9/4/2009,* in both of the Date From Range boxes.

6. Click the box at the bottom of the window to show the accounts receivable totals at the end of the report.

7. Press the OK button.

8. Review both pages of the report.

9. Close the Preview Report window.

Analysis Reports

Several reports can be prepared with the NDCMedisoft™ program that are useful in analyzing a medical practice's financial activity. These reports include the Billing/Payment Status and Practice Analysis reports. Each report provides a different perspective of the financial data stored in the patient accounting system.

Billing/Payment Status Report

The **Billing/Payment Status report** is an excellent practice management tool. It lists the status of all transactions that have a responsible insurance carrier, showing who has paid and who has not been billed (see Figure 7-4 on page 120). This information is helpful in determining whether billing charges can be applied to a patient balance.

The report is sorted by Chart Number and then Case. Every chart number listed shows a patient balance and whether there have been any unapplied payments or unapplied adjustments.

Billing/Payment Status Report
As of September 7, 2009

Date	Document	Procedure	Amount	Policy 1	Policy 2	Policy 3	Guarantor	Adjustments	Balance
BAREL000	Ellen Barmenstein (614)274-4242								
Case 1	1: Blue Cross/Blue Shield (614)241-9000								
8/28/2009	0508290000	99212	44.00	-35.20*	0.00*	0.00*	9/7/2009	0.00*	8.80
							SubTotal:		8.80
						Unapplied Payments and Adjustments:			0.00
							Case Balance:		8.80
Case 29	1: Blue Cross/Blue Shield (614)241-9000								
9/4/2009	0407250000	99211	30.00	0.00*	0.00*	0.00*	9/7/2009	0.00*	30.00
9/4/2009	0407250000	90471	10.00	-8.00*	0.00*	0.00*	9/7/2009	0.00*	2.00
9/4/2009	0407250000	90658	12.00	-9.60*	0.00*	0.00*	9/7/2009	0.00*	2.40
							SubTotal:		34.40
						Unapplied Payments and Adjustments:			0.00
							Case Balance:		34.40
							Patient Balance:		43.20
BELSA001	Sarina Bell (614)241-6124								
Case 32	1: U.S. Life (800)921-6320								
9/4/2009	0407250000	99212	39.60	Not Billed	0.00*	0.00*	Not Billed	0.00*	39.60
9/4/2009	0407250000	87430	28.80	Not Billed	0.00*	0.00*	Not Billed	0.00*	28.80
9/4/2009	0407250000	85025	22.50	Not Billed	0.00*	0.00*	Not Billed	0.00*	22.50
							SubTotal:		90.90
						Unapplied Payments and Adjustments:			0.00
							Case Balance:		90.90
							Patient Balance:		90.90
FELST000	Stanley Feldman (614)555-9295								
Case 6	1: Blue Cross/Blue Shield (614)241-9000								
7/28/2009	0507280000	93015	325.00	-260.00*	0.00*	0.00*	Not Billed	0.00*	65.00

Printed on 9/7/2009 12:58:48 PM   This program is registered to   Page 1
* Indicates that this payment is complete   MCGRAW-HILL TEXTBOOK USE ONLY
A date in the payment columns indicates the billing date

Figure 7-4 *Sample Page from a Billing/Payment Status Report*

Family Care Center
Practice Analysis
From September 1, 2009 to September 30, 2009

Code	Modifier	Description	Amount	Units	Average	Cost	Net
02		Patient payment, check	-60.00	1	-60.00	0.00	-60.00
82465		Cholesterol test	21.00	1	21.00	0.00	21.00
85025	90	CBC w/diff	22.50	1	22.50	0.00	22.50
87430		Strep screen	28.80	1	28.80	0.00	28.80
90471		Immunization administration	20.00	2	10.00	0.00	20.00
90658		Influenza injection, older than 3	12.00	1	12.00	0.00	12.00
90707		MMR immunization	105.00	1	105.00	0.00	105.00
99204		OF--New patient, moderate	147.00	1	147.00	0.00	147.00
99211		OF--Established patient, minimal	30.00	1	30.00	0.00	30.00
99212		OF--Established patient, low	151.20	4	37.80	0.00	151.20
99383		Preventive new, 5-11 years	140.00	1	140.00	0.00	140.00
BCBPAY		Blue Cross Blue Shield Payment	-628.00	11	-57.09	0.00	-628.00
TRICOC		Tricare Copayment Charge	10.00	1	10.00	0.00	10.00
TRICOP		Tricare Patient Copayment	-10.00	1	-10.00	0.00	-10.00
USLCOC		USLife Copayment Charge	30.00	2	15.00	0.00	30.00
USLCOP		USLife Patient Copayment	-30.00	2	-15.00	0.00	-30.00

Figure 7-5 *Sample Page from a Practice Analysis Report*

Practice Analysis Report

The **Practice Analysis report** shows the total revenue for each procedure performed during a specific period (such as a week, month, or year). The summary section of the report includes information such as total procedure charges, total insurance payments, total patient payments, and net effect on accounts receivable. This report (see Figure 7-5) is useful in analyzing which procedures generated the most revenue. Subsequently, the report can be used to perform a profitability analysis and may be helpful to an accountant when preparing financial statements for the medical practice.

Computer Practice 7-3: *Printing a Practice Analysis Report*

1. Select the option to print a Practice Analysis report.

2. Choose to preview the report on your screen.

3. Enter *9/1/2009* in the first Date From Range field and *9/30/2009* in the second Date From Range field.

4. Click the box at the bottom of the window to show the accounts receivable totals. Then press the OK button.

5. Review the information provided. Notice there are two pages. Do not print this report, unless instructed otherwise.

6. Close the Preview Report window.

Family Care Center

Patient Aging

From January 1, 2009 to September 30, 2009

Chart	Name	Birthdate	Current 0 - 30	Past 31 - 60	Past 61 - 90	Past 91 --->	Total Balance
BAREL000	Ellen Barmenstein	10/16/1982	34.40	8.80			43.20
Last Pmt: -9.60	On: 9/7/2009	(614)274-4242					
BELSA001	Sarina Bell	1/21/1999	90.90				90.90
Last Pmt: -15.00	On: 9/4/2009	(614)241-6124					
FELST000	Stanley Feldman	1/30/1959			65.00		65.00
Last Pmt: -260.00	On: 9/7/2009	(614)555-9295					
JOHMA000	Marion Johnson	10/15/1956		4.20	57.00		61.20
Last Pmt: -16.80	On: 9/7/2009	(614)726-9898					
JONEL000	Elizabeth Jones	8/26/1974	39.60				39.60
Last Pmt: -15.00	On: 9/4/2009	(614)321-5555					
LOMCE000	Cedera Lomos	5/21/1957	147.00				147.00
Last Pmt: 0.00	On:	(614)221-0202					
LOMLI000	Lisa Lomos	6/3/2004	255.00				255.00
Last Pmt: 0.00	On:	(614)221-0202					
MITHE000	Herbert Mitchell	10/8/1934		7.80			7.80
Last Pmt: -31.20	On: 8/31/2009	(614)861-0909					
PATLE000	Leila Patterson	2/14/1949	65.00				65.00
Last Pmt: 0.00	On:	(614)626-2099					
PETAN000	Ann Peterson	10/12/1961			32.00		32.00
Last Pmt: -10.00	On: 7/20/2009	(614)555-8989					
PETPE000	Peter Peterson	8/8/1958				77.00	77.00
Last Pmt: -10.00	On: 6/12/2009	(614)555-2929					
SMIJA000	James L Smith	11/27/1978		8.80	8.80		17.60
Last Pmt: -35.20	On: 9/7/2009	(614)879-2521					
TANHI000	Hiro Tanaka	6/10/2000	28.00	83.00			111.00
Last Pmt: -10.00	On: 9/4/2009	(614)751-7732					
WONJO000	Jo Wong	9/6/1939			325.00		325.00
Last Pmt: 0.00	On:	(614)751-7677					
WONLI000	Li Yu Wong	12/13/1937		5.60			5.60
Last Pmt: -22.40	On: 8/31/2009	(614)751-7677					
	Report Aging Totals		$659.90	$118.20	$487.80	$77.00	1,342.90
	Percent of Aging Total		49.1%	8.8%	36.3%	5.7%	100.00%

Figure 7-6 *Sample Page from a Patient Aging Report*

Aging Reports

Aging is the classification of accounts receivables by the amount of time they are past due. A **Patient Aging report,** for example, shows the "age" for all outstanding patient charges. The report classifies charges using four aging categories—Current (0–30 days), 31–60 days, 61–90 days, and 91 days or older. See the sample Patient Aging report shown in Figure 7-6. The Patient Aging report is an important tool in collections since you can easily identify patients whose accounts are past due.

Primary Insurance Aging

As of 9/30/2009

Date of Service	Procedure	-- Past -- 0 - 30	-- Past -- 31 - 60	-- Past -- 61 - 90	-- Past -- 91 - 120	-- Past -- 121 --->	Total Balance
TRICARE (3)							**(614)241-8080**

PETPE000   Peter Peterson   SS: 238-83-8392   Policy: 138838392   Group: 1456
Birthdate: 8/8/1958
Claim: 3   Initial Billing Date: 9/4/2009   Last Billing Date: 9/4/2009

Date of Service	Procedure	0 - 30	31 - 60	61 - 90	91 - 120	121 --->	Total Balance
6/12/2009	99212	28.00	0.00	0.00	0.00	0.00	28.00
6/12/2009	73090	28.00	0.00	0.00	0.00	0.00	28.00
6/12/2009	90703	13.00	0.00	0.00	0.00	0.00	13.00
6/12/2009	90471	8.00	0.00	0.00	0.00	0.00	8.00
		$77.00	$0.00	$0.00	$0.00	$0.00	$77.00
	Insurance Totals	$77.00	$0.00	$0.00	$0.00	$0.00	$77.00
	Report Aging Totals	$77.00	$0.00	$0.00	$0.00	$0.00	$77.00
	Percent of Aging Total	100.00 %	0.00%	0.00%	0.00%	0.00%	100.00%

Figure 7-7   *Sample Page from a Primary Insurance Aging Report*

An **Insurance Aging report** is an excellent tool for tracking claims filed with insurance carriers. There are three insurance aging reports: Primary Insurance Aging, Secondary Insurance Aging, and Tertiary Insurance Aging. These reports provide aging information similar to the Patient Aging report. Instead of patients, however, the reports show each insurance carrier and its outstanding balance status (see Figure 7-7).

Computer Practice 7-4: *Printing a Patient Aging Report*

1. Select the option to print a Patient Aging report.

2. Choose to preview the report on your screen.

3. Enter *1/1/2009* in the first Date From Range field and *9/30/2009* in the second Date From Range field. Then press the OK button.

4. Review the information provided. Do not print this report, unless instructed otherwise.

5. Close the Preview Report window.

Collection Reports

NDCMedisoft™ provides a number of collection reports that can be used to locate overdue patient or insurance accounts.

Patient Collection Report

9/30/2009

Statement Number	Initial Bill Date	Last Bill Date	Last Patient Pay Date	Last Patient Pay Amount	Submission	Statement Type	Statement Total
BAREL000- Ellen Barmenstein			Phone: (614)274-4242				
1	9/7/2009	9/7/2009			1	Remainder	$43.20
							$43.20
						Total:	$43.20

Figure 7-8 *Sample Page from a Patient Collection Report*

Patient Collection Report

The **Patient Collection report** makes it easy to identify outstanding balances, helping you manage your patient collections. The report draws information from the Statement Management area of the program and includes information such as number, patient name, telephone number, Statement Number, Initial Bill Date, Last Bill Date, Last Patient Payment Date, and Last Patient Payment Amount. A sample Patient Collection report is illustrated in Figure 7-8.

Insurance Collection Reports

Insurance Collection reports are similar to the Patient Collection reports, except that the listings are for insurance carriers instead of patients. **Insurance Collection reports** are used to monitor outstanding claim balances. The report is based on information in the Claim Management area of the program and provides details such as the Claim Number, Chart Number, and Primary (Secondary, Tertiary) Bill Date for each payer. Figure 7-9 shows a sample Insurance Collection report.

The selections for the report can be filtered by Chart Number Range, Date Created Range, Insurance Carrier 1 Range (or 2 or 3 for secondary and tertiary claims), Initial Billing Date 1 Range (or 2 or 3 for secondary and tertiary claims), and Claim Status 1 Match (or 2 or 3 for secondary and tertiary claims).

Computer Practice 7-5: *Printing an Insurance Collection Report*

1. Select the option to print a Primary Insurance Collection report.

2. Choose to preview the report on your screen.

3. Leave the default entries in the Data Selection Questions dialog box as they are. Then press the OK button.

4. Review the information provided. Do not print this report, unless instructed otherwise.

5. Close the Preview Report window.

Primary Insurance Collection Report

9/7/2009

Claim	Chart	Primary Bill Date	Batch 1	Date Created	Submission Count	Claim Total
1 - Medicare				**Phone: (215)599-0205**		
14	WONJO000		0	7/31/2009	0	$325.00
					Total:	$325.00
10 - U.S. Life				**Phone: (800)921-6320**		
30	BELSA001		0	9/4/2009	0	$90.90
31	JONEL000		0	9/4/2009	0	$39.60
					Total:	$130.50
13 - Oxford				**Phone: (614)555-0014**		
35	PATLE000		0	9/4/2009	0	$65.00
					Total:	$65.00
3 - TRICARE				**Phone: (614)241-8080**		
3	PETPE000	9/4/2009	1	6/12/2009	1	$87.00
12	PETAN000		0	7/24/2009	0	$42.00
18	TANHI000		0	8/14/2009	0	$55.00
22	TANHI000		0	8/21/2009	0	$28.00
36	TANHI000		0	9/4/2009	0	$28.00
					Total:	$240.00
4 - Blue Cross/Blue Shield				**Phone: (614)241-9000**		
5	MITCA000		0	6/19/2009	0	$60.00
29	BAREL000		0	9/4/2009	0	$52.00
32	LOMCE000		0	9/4/2009	0	$147.00
33	LOMLI000		0	9/4/2009	0	$140.00
34	LOMLI000		0	9/4/2009	0	$115.00
					Total:	$514.00
					Report Total:	$1,274.50

Figure 7-9 *Sample Page from an Insurance Collection Report*

Patient Ledgers

The **Patient Ledger report** lets you view the account activity for each patient (see Figure 7-10 on page 126). The ledger includes the procedure charges, payments, and adjustments for all patients or selected patients. It also shows the current balance and any unpaid charges.

Family Care Center
Patient Account Ledger
As of September 7, 2009

Entry	Date	POS	Description	Procedure	Document	Provider	Amount
BAREL000		**Ellen Barmenstein**		(614)274-4242			
	Last Payment: -9.60	On: 9/7/2009					
86	8/28/2009			99212	0508290000	1	44.00
205	9/4/2009			99211	0407250000	1	30.00
206	9/4/2009			90471	0407250000	1	10.00
207	9/4/2009			90658	0407250000	1	12.00
227	9/7/2009		#3574896 Blue Cross/Blue Shiel	BCBPAY	0508290000	1	-35.20
228	9/7/2009		#3574896 Blue Cross/Blue Shiel	BCBPAY	0407250000	1	0.00
229	9/7/2009		#3574896 Blue Cross/Blue Shiel	BCBPAY	0407250000	1	-8.00
230	9/7/2009		#3574896 Blue Cross/Blue Shiel	BCBPAY	0407250000	1	-9.60
	Patient Totals						43.20
BELSA001		**Sarina Bell**		(614)241-6124			
	Last Payment: -15.00	On: 9/4/2009					
214	9/4/2009			99212	0407250000	1	39.60
215	9/4/2009			87430	0407250000	1	28.80
216	9/4/2009			85025	0407250000	1	22.50
217	9/4/2009			USLCOC	0407250000	1	15.00
218	9/4/2009			USLCOP	0407250000	1	-15.00
	Patient Totals						90.90
FELST000		**Stanley Feldman**		(614)555-9295			
	Last Payment: -260.00	On: 9/7/2009					
83	7/28/2009			93015	0507280000	1	325.00
220	9/7/2009		#36094251 Blue Cross/Blue Shie	BCBPAY	0507280000	1	-260.00
	Patient Totals						65.00
JOHMA000		**Marion Johnson**		(614)726-9898			
	Last Payment: -16.80	On: 9/7/2009					
75	7/15/2009			93000	0507150000	1	70.00
74	7/15/2009			99215	0507150000	1	135.00
77	8/18/2009			82947	0508180000	1	21.00
76	7/15/2009			71010	0507150000	1	80.00
221	9/7/2009		#36094251 Blue Cross/Blue Shie	BCBPAY	0507150000	1	-108.00
222	9/7/2009		#36094251 Blue Cross/Blue Shie	BCBPAY	0507150000	1	-56.00
223	9/7/2009		#36094251 Blue Cross/Blue Shie	BCBPAY	0507150000	1	-64.00
224	9/7/2009		#36094251 Blue Cross/Blue Shie	BCBPAY	0508180000	1	-16.80
	Patient Totals						61.20
JONEL000		**Elizabeth Jones**		(614)321-5555			
	Last Payment: -15.00	On: 9/4/2009					
102	8/28/2009			99212	0508290000	1	39.60
103	8/28/2009			90471	0508290000	1	9.00
172	8/28/2009			90703	0407190000	1	18.00
144	8/28/2009			USLCOP	0407190000	1	-15.00
173	8/28/2009			USLCOC	0407190000	1	15.00

Figure 7-10 *Sample Page from a Patient Ledger Report*

1. Pull down the Reports menu and choose the Patient Ledger option.

2. Choose to preview the report on the screen.

3. The program displays the Data Selection Questions dialog box (see Figure 7-11). As with the Data Selection Questions dialog boxes for other reports, the options let you customize the report to display only the data you need. For example, if all the fields are blank, the program prints a report using all of the data stored in the database. However, you could print a Patient Ledger report for only one patient by entering that patient's chart number in the Chart Number Range fields. Or you could print a report for a specific time period. In this case, you will print a report that includes data for all patients as of September 4, 2009.

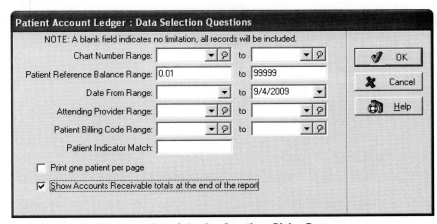

Figure 7-11 *Patient Ledger Data Selection Questions Dialog Box*

4. In the second Date From Range box, delete the default entry and enter *9/4/2009.*

5. Click the box labeled Show Accounts Receivable Totals at the End of the Report.

6. Press the OK button.

7. Zoom the report (pages 1–3), and review the information shown for the Family Care Center's patients.

8. Print the report, and then close the Preview Report window.

List Reports

As you are aware, NDCMedisoft™ stores most of the data for a medical practice in various databases. The data can be printed as lists—procedure lists, diagnosis lists, patient lists, insurance carrier lists, and so on. You can use the Custom Report List option on the Reports menu to access the list reports.

1. Pull down the Reports menu, and choose Custom Report List.

2. The Open Report dialog box appears. Click on the List radio button to show only the list reports (see Figure 7-12.)

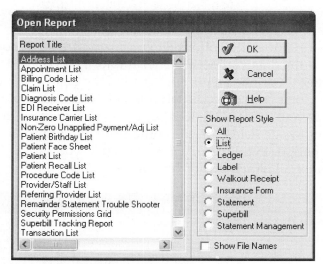

Figure 7-12 *Open Report Dialog Box*

3. Select the Procedure Code List option, and then click the OK button.

4. Choose to display the list on the screen.

5. Leave all fields blank in the Data Selection Questions dialog box, and press the OK button.

6. Review the procedures shown on the report. Close the Preview Report window.

7. Using the same procedure, display a patient list of all patients. Close the Preview Report window.

8. Display any of the other lists if you are interested in the information they contain.

Designing Custom Reports and Bills

You can generate numerous reports using the NDCMedisoft™ program. However, you may want to customize a report to meet a particular need. For example, you could design a special report to be sent to an insurance carrier. In these instances, you can use the NDCMedisoft™ Report Designer to modify an existing report or create a completely new report (see Figure 7-13). The Report Designer is a very powerful tool that provides all the features you need to prepare a new report layout.

Although this tutorial does not cover the Report Designer, you can explore this option on your own. To access the Report Designer, choose the Design Custom Reports and Bills option from the Reports menu. Remember that you can use the help system to learn more about the Report Designer if you have any questions.

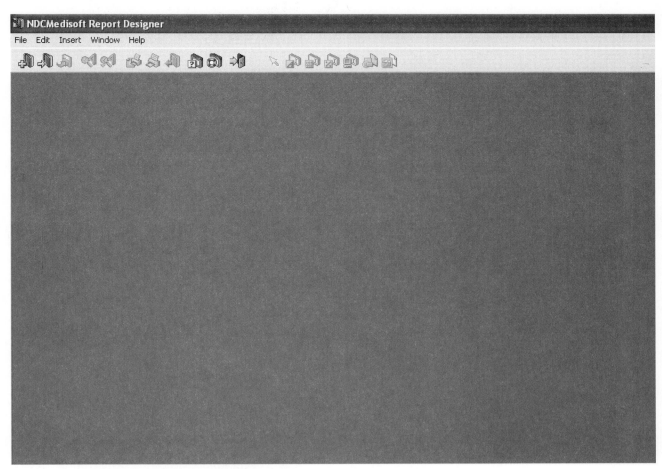

Figure 7-13   *Main Window of NDCMedisoft™ Report Designer*

✓CHECKPOINT

1. Which report lists each patient account and identifies the amount of time each account has been past due?

2. Which report shows the total revenue for each procedure?

3. Which report creates a list of all procedure codes in the database?

4. Which report includes information organized by patient and is typically printed at the end of each day?

Computer Practice 7-8: *Exiting the Program and Making a Backup Copy*

Practice quitting the software and making a backup copy of your work by following these steps:

1. Choose Exit from the File menu, or use the toolbar to select this option.

2. Insert your working copy of the Student Data Disk in Drive A:.

3. Click the Back Up Data Now button.

4. In the Destination File Path and Name box, enter *A:\PBChap7.mbk.*

5. Click the Start Backup button. When the Backup Complete box appears, click OK. The NDCMedisoft™ program shuts down.

6. Remove the floppy disk from Drive A:.

7. Store your disk in a safe place.

Chapter 7 Review

Define the Terms

Write a definition for each term: (Obj. 7-1)

1. Aging

   _____

2. Billing/Payment Status report

   _____

3. Cash flow

   _____

4. Insurance Aging report

   _____

5. Insurance Collection reports

   _____

6. Patient Aging report

   _____

7. Patient Collection report

   _____

8. Patient Ledger report

   _____

9. Payables

   _____

10. Practice Analysis report

    _____

11. Receivables

    _____

CHECK YOUR UNDERSTANDING

12. Does the NDCMedisoft™ program let you set up filters to print only selected information on a report? Explain. (Obj. 7-2)

_____

13. Describe how you can use the controls in the Preview Report window to review the information on a report. (Obj. 7-2)

_____

14. How do the Patient and Procedure Day Sheet reports differ? (Obj. 7-3)

_____

_____

15. Describe how the Billing/Payment Status report can be used. (Obj. 7-4)

_____

16. If you were asked to print a report for all patients with outstanding balances, including the length of time each account has been unpaid, what report would you print? (Obj. 7-5)

_____

17. What information is included on the Patient Collection report? (Obj. 7-6)

_____

18. What information is included on the Patient Ledger report? (Obj. 7-7)

_____

19. Describe the various list reports available in NDCMedisoft™. (Obj. 7-8)

_____

20. List several reasons why you might need to use the NDCMedisoft™ Report Designer to customize a report. (Obj. 7-9)

_____

CRITICAL ANALYSIS EXERCISE

21. Why is the information on a Patient Aging report or an Insurance Aging report so valuable in monitoring accounts receivable data? (Obj. 7-5)

_____

_____

Family Care Center: A Patient Billing Simulation

Now that you have completed the tutorial, you are ready to begin the patient billing simulation using the NDCMedisoft™ program. As the new billing assistant for the Family Care Center, your job is to process the patient billing for the medical practice. The simulation takes place from Monday, November 2, 2009 through Friday, November 6, 2009. Tuesday, November 3 is Election Day and the office is closed.

As you complete the simulation, you may notice that the volume of work is not the same as you would expect in an actual medical practice. However, the tasks you will perform are similar to those a billing assistant would perform on a daily basis.

Before you begin, review the Office Procedures Manual shown below on pages 133 through 135. Then, refer to the step-by-step instructions for the individual days that follow on pages 135 through 140 to complete the simulation. If you need assistance using the software, refer to the tutorial or use the Help information built into the software.

Office Procedures Manual

Review the office procedures for the Family Care Center. Some of these tasks are already completed for you, but in an actual office, you would perform each of these duties.

Daily Tasks Before Patients Arrive

- Assist receptionist in completing an encounter form for each patient with a scheduled appointment. Fill in the patient's name, address, chart number, and the date.
- Gather the materials for the day: NDCMedisoft™ data disk, Friday afternoon's encounter forms, and any receipts (cash or checks) from the previous day. The receptionist keeps the receipts in a locked drawer overnight.
- Prepare a change fund for the receptionist.
- Turn on the computer and start NDCMedisoft™.

Morning Tasks

Each morning you must enter the transactions and payments from the previous afternoon, and then prepare a bank deposit slip. Deposits are usually made at noon.

- Enter the transaction data from the previous afternoon.
- If necessary, update any patient accounts.
- Open the mail and record each check received. Enter the payment amount and the check number. Indicate whether the payment is from an insurer or a patient. Apply the payments to patient accounts.
- Review electronic funds transfers and enter the payment information in NDCMedisoft™.
- Prepare a bank deposit slip for the checks received in the mail and for receipts on hand from the previous day.
- Print a patient day sheet for the previous day.
- Give the day sheets to the office manager and take the deposit to the bank.

Afternoon Tasks

During the afternoon, your primary task is to enter the patient information, charges, and payments for those patients who had morning appointments. Other tasks include transmitting claims for the previous day's transactions.

- Create and send insurance claims for the previous day's visits.
- Gather the Patient Information Forms for the new patients who had morning appointments, and enter this information into the system.
- Update any information for established patients.
- Using the encounter forms provided by the receptionist, enter the data for patients seen in the morning.
- Time permitting, enter the transactions for the afternoon appointments.
- Back up the patient billing data.

Other Tasks During the Day

- Respond to calls from patients about their accounts.
- Relieve the receptionist when needed.
- Make collection calls to patients and insurers.
- Call insurers about managed-care cases as needed.
- Fill out (or print) special forms for disability and so forth.

Weekly Tasks

- On Friday, print a Patient Aging report and consult with the office manager regarding any overdue accounts. If necessary, contact patients concerning past due account balances. Write off bad debts after consulting with the office manager. (Typically, these are for charges more than a year old where there is no chance of collecting from the patient or insurer.)

- On Friday afternoons, prepare the appropriate patient remainder statements:
  - 1st Friday—Patients A-L
  - 3rd Friday—Patients M-Z
- Print a Practice Analysis report.

Monday, November 2, 2009

1. Remove Source Documents 19 through 30 on pages 189–211. Review the information provided on the source documents before entering data.

2. Start the NDCMedisoft™ program.

3. Set the program date to October 30, 2009. The patient transactions from Friday afternoon, October 30, have not been recorded yet.

4. Record these transactions from last Friday using the information provided on Source Documents 19-23. Use the Enter Transactions option to record the procedure charges and patient payments. Use the Enter Deposits/Payments option to record insurance carrier payments. Print a walkout receipt for each patient who makes a payment.

   - Use the encounter form for Janine Bell (Source Document 19) to record the procedure charge and payment.

     First you will need to create a new case. Remember to enter the Price Code in the Account tab and to select Herbert Bell as Guarantor in the Personal tab. When completing the Policy 1 tab, you need to know that Janine is covered by her husband's policy from U.S. Life (Policy #: 50632, Group #: 6209, Price Code B, $15 copayment). Dr. Yan accepts assignment from U.S. Life, which pays 100% of services (Box A through Box H).

     Apply the payment and print a walkout receipt.

   - Enter the information to record the procedure charge for Felix Suarez (Source Document 20).

     Create a new case for this office visit. You will need to review an earlier case to get the necessary policy information. Or, you can copy the existing case, and then change the description and diagnosis.

     Apply the payment and print a walkout receipt.

   - Record the two procedure charges and payment written on Sarah Fitzwilliams's encounter form (Source Document 21).

     To begin, create a new case. Sarah is a full-time student covered by her father's TRICARE insurance (Policy #: 457091, Group #: 3265, Price Code C, $10 copayment). Dr. Yan accepts assignment from TRICARE, which pays 100% of services (Box A through Box H).

     Print a walkout receipt.

- Enter the information from the encounter form for Marion Johnson (Source Document 22). Use the existing case but add an additional diagnosis.

5. A remittance advice that was received last Friday has not been processed. The information you need to record these payments is provided on Source Document 23. Enter these payment transactions. Be sure that the program date is set to 10/30/2009. Also, for the purposes of this simulation, make sure the Sort By field is set to Claim Number.

6. Print a patient day sheet for Friday, October 30, 2009. Delete the dates in the Date Created Range boxes and enter October 30, 2009 in both Date From Range boxes. Be sure to check the box to show accounts receivable data at the end of the report.

7. Verify that you have entered the information correctly. The total receipts on hand should be $361.60. If the amounts match, continue with the next step. Otherwise, find your error, correct it, and print updated reports. After verifying the amounts, you would complete a bank deposit slip and take the deposit to the bank.

8. Create the insurance claim forms for the patient charges you just entered. Use 10/30/2009 to create claim forms for that date only. Most offices, including Family Care Center, transmit claims electronically. However, it is not possible to actually transmit claims in this simulation. Therefore, we will assume they have been transmitted electronically once they have been created. Along these lines, for the purposes of this simulation, you will need to manually change the status of claims from Ready to Send to Sent.

9. Change the program date to November 2, 2009, since you will now begin entering some of today's transactions.

10. Set up patient accounts for two patients who had appointments with Dr. Yan this morning. Mr. and Mrs. Andrews will need to be entered as new patients. Use the Patient Information Forms shown in Source Documents 24 and 25 to record the patient information. Then create cases for both patients.

11. Update the patient information for James Smith (Source Document 26).

12. Enter the procedure charges and payments for the patients who had appointments this morning—Darla Andrews, Bill Andrews, Cedera Lomos, and Stanley Feldman (Source Documents 27-30). Print a walkout receipt for each patient who makes a payment. Be sure that the program date is set to Monday (11/02/2009) when you record the transactions.

Notes: (a) Use the existing case for Cedera Lomos since the reason for this visit is the same as the last visit. (b) Create a new case for Stanley Feldman's visit.

13. Exit the NDCMedisoft™ program.

14. Make a backup copy of your work.

Tuesday, November 3, 2009

Office closed for Election Day.

Wednesday, November 4, 2009

1. Remove Source Documents 31 through 42 on pages 213–235. Review the information provided on the source documents.

2. Start the NDCMedisoft™ program.

3. Set the program date to November 2, 2009 before entering the transactions from Monday afternoon. The office was closed Tuesday, November 3, for Election Day.

4. Record the following transactions from Monday using the information provided on Source Documents 31-34. Use the Enter Transactions option to record the procedure charges and payments. Print a walkout receipt for each patient who makes a payment.

   - Enter the procedure charges and payment for Ethan Sampson (Source Document 31).

     Create a new case. Ethan is a full-time college student, covered by his mother's (Caroline Sampson) insurance (U.S. Life, Policy #: 0123456, Group #: R123, Price Code B, $15 copayment). Dr. Yan accepts assignment from U.S. Life, which pays 100% of services (Box A through Box H).

     Remember to enter 11/2/2009 for the transaction date and print a walkout receipt.

   - Enter the information and record the transactions for Jo Black, who is a new patient (Source Documents 32 and 33). Dr. Yan accepts assignment from Blue Cross/Blue Shield, which pays 80% of services (Box A through Box H). Jo has met her deductible.

   - Create a new case and record the transactions for Sarina Bell. Be sure to enter and apply the copayment and print a walkout receipt (Source Document 34).

5. A patient, James Smith, called the office to inquire about his account balance. Write the patient's account balance in the space provided. BALANCE: $_____.

6. Process the remittance advice received Monday, November 2 (Source Document 35).

7. Print a patient day sheet for Monday, November 2, 2009. Delete the dates in the Date Created Range boxes and enter November 2, 2009 in both Date From Range boxes. Be sure to check the box to show accounts receivable data at the end of the report.

8. Verify that you have entered the information correctly. The receipts total $203.00. If this amount does not match the information on the reports, find the error and make the necessary correction.

9. Create the insurance claim forms for the patient charges you just entered. Change the status of claims from Ready to Send to Sent.

10. Change the program date to November 4, 2009 to enter today's transactions.

11. Process the transactions from this morning (Source Documents 36-42). Remember to print a walkout receipt for each patient who makes a payment.

    - Enter the transactions for John Gardiner (Source Document 36).

      Create a new case. Gardiner's health insurance carrier is Physician's Choice (Policy #: 6397008, Group #: J10-32, Price Code B, $15 copayment). Dr. Yan accepts assignment from Physician's Choice, which pays 100% of services (Box A through Box H).

    - Record the new telephone number for Paul Ramos (Source Document 37).

    - Input the new patient information and create a new case for Sam Wu (Source Documents 38 and 39). Remember to complete the Condition tab in the Case folder since this visit is for an automobile accident.

      Enter the procedures and copayment. Print a walkout receipt.

    - Enter the transactions for Paul Ramos.

      First, create a new case. Ramos is a full-time student, single, and currently not employed (Source Document 40). He is covered by his mother's health insurance. Maritza Ramos and her son are insured with Physician's Choice (Policy #: 33246A, Group #: EF719, Price Code B, $15 copayment). As you already know, Dr. Yan accepts assignment from Physician's Choice, which pays 100% of services (Box A through Box H).

    - Record the procedure charges for Ellen Barmenstein (Source Document 41).

      Be sure to enter a new case for this visit.

    - Record the procedure charge and payment for Elizabeth Jones (Source Document 42). This visit is related to the previous Laceration case.

12. Exit the NDCMedisoft™ program, and make a backup copy of your work.

Thursday, November 5, 2009

1. Remove and review Source Documents 43 through 50 on pages 237–251.

2. Start the NDCMedisoft™ program.

3. Set the program date to November 4, 2009 to enter the transactions from Wednesday afternoon.

4. Record the following transactions from Wednesday using the information provided on Source Documents 43-46. Print a walkout receipt for each patient.

   - Enter the procedure charges for James Smith (Source Document 43).

   - Record the transactions for Joe Abate, a new patient (Source Documents 44 and 45).

   - Record the procedure charge for Sarabeth Smith (Source Document 46).

   Sarabeth, who is single, has her own insurance policy with Blue Cross Blue Shield (Policy #: 03467, Group #: 2450, Price Code A, $250 Deductible). Dr. Yan accepts assignment from Blue Cross Blue Shield, which pays 80% of services (Box A through Box H). Sarabeth has met her deductible for 2009.

5. A patient, Jo Black, called the office to inquire about her account balance. Write the patient's total account balance in the space provided.
   TOTAL BALANCE: $_____.

   Since she has met her deductible, what amount of the balance is she responsible for? Write that in the space provided.
   HER RESPONSIBILITY: $_____.

6. Process the check from Marion Johnson that was received yesterday (Source Document 47).

7. Print a patient day sheet for Wednesday, November 4, 2009. Delete the dates in the Date Created Range boxes and enter November 4, 2009 in both Date From Range boxes. Be sure to check the box to show accounts receivable data at the end of the report.

8. Verify that you have entered the information correctly so that you can prepare a bank deposit slip. The cash and checks on hand should total $136.20. Make any necessary corrections.

9. Create the insurance claim forms for the patient charges. Be sure to change the status of newly created claims.

10. Change the program date to November 5, 2009 to enter today's transactions.

11. Process the transactions from this morning (Source Documents 48-50). Remember to print a walkout receipt for each patient.

    - Enter the transactions for Maritza Ramos (Source Document 48).

      Create a new case. Maritza is a full-time employee of Sara's Dresses. You will need to look at her son Paul's case to locate the insurance information.

      Enter the charges and copayment and print a walkout receipt.

    - Create a new case and then record the procedure charge and payment for Sarina Bell (Source Document 49).

    - Record the transactions for Jo Wong (Source Document 50).

12. Exit the NDCMedisoft™ program, and make a backup copy of your work.

Friday, November 6, 2009

1. Remove and review Source Documents 51 through 55b on pages 253–263.

2. Start the NDCMedisoft™ program.

3. Set the program date to November 5, 2009 to enter the transactions from Thursday afternoon.

4. Process the check from James L. Smith that was received yesterday (Source Document 51).

5. Print a patient day sheet for Thursday, November 5, 2009. Delete the dates in the Date Created Range boxes, and enter November 5, 2009 in both Date From Range boxes. Be sure to check the box to show accounts receivable data at the end of the report.

6. Verify that you have entered the information correctly so that you can prepare a bank deposit slip. The checks on hand total $47.60. Make any necessary corrections.

7. Create the insurance claim forms for the patient charges. Change the status of the new claims to Sent.

8. Change the program date to November 6, 2009 to enter today's transactions.

9. Process the transactions from this morning (Source Documents 52-54). Remember to print walkout receipts for patients who make payments.

    *   Enter the procedure charges for Surendra Uzwahl, a new patient (Source Documents 52 and 53).

    *   Record the transactions for Jonathan Bell (Source Document 54). He is a full-time student, covered by his father's (Herbert Bell) insurance.

10. Record and apply the payment from Blue Cross Blue Shield (Source Documents 55a and 55b).

11. Create remainder statements for patients whose last names begin with A through L. For the purposes of this simulation, set the Sort By field in the Statement Management window to Statement Number. Do not enter a date range filter when you print the statements. All date boxes should be empty (you may need to delete default data).

12. Change the status of all Batch 0 statements from Ready to Send to Sent.

13. Print a patient aging report for all patients. Leave the first Date From Range box blank, and enter November 6, 2009 in the second box.

14. Print a Practice Analysis report. Use 10/30/2009 through 11/6/2009 for the report Date From range. Check the box to show accounts receivable data.

15. Exit the NDCMedisoft™ program, and make a backup copy of your work.

16. Complete the Simulation Assessment Test if your instructor provided you with a copy of this test. Use the reports you printed this session to answer the questions on the test.

Appendix: Office Hours

WHAT YOU NEED TO KNOW

To use this appendix, you need to know how to:

- Start NDCMedisoft™, use menus, and enter and edit text.
- Work with chart numbers and codes.

WHAT YOU WILL LEARN

In this appendix, you will learn how to:

- Start Office Hours.
- View the appointment schedule.
- Enter an appointment.
- Change or delete an appointment.
- Move or copy an appointment.

Introduction to Office Hours

Appointment scheduling is one of the most important tasks in a medical office. Different medical procedures take different lengths of time, and each appointment must be the right length. On the one hand, physicians want to be able to go from one appointment to another without unnecessary breaks. On the other hand, patients should not be kept waiting more than a few minutes for a physician. Managing and juggling the schedule is usually the job of a medical office assistant working at the front desk. NDCMedisoft™ provides a special program called Office Hours to handle appointment scheduling.

Overview of the Office Hours Window

The Office Hours program has its own window (see Figure A-1 on page 142) including its own menu bar and toolbar. The Office Hours menu bar lists the menus available: File, Edit, View, Lists, Reports, Tools, and Help. Under the menu bar is a toolbar with shortcut buttons. The functions of Office Hours are accessed by selecting a choice from one of the menus or by clicking a button on the toolbar.

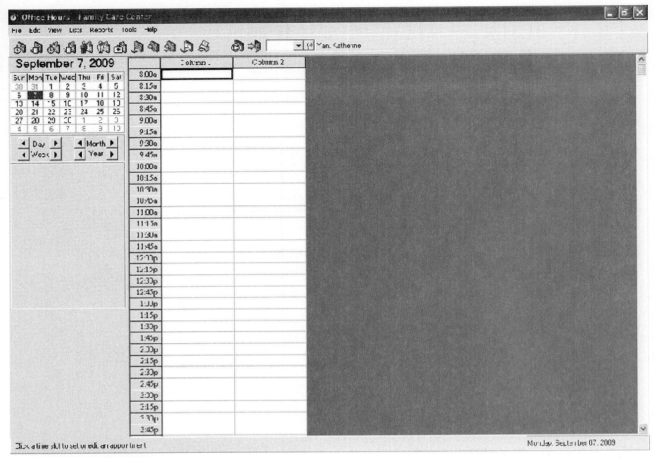

Figure A-1   *Office Hours Window*

Located just below the menu bar, the toolbar contains a series of buttons that represent the most common activities performed in Office Hours. These buttons are shortcuts for frequently used menu commands. The toolbar displays 14 buttons.

The left half of the Office Hours screen displays the current date and a calendar of the current month. The current date is highlighted on the calendar. When a different date is clicked on the calendar, the calendar switches to the new date. TAKE NOTE: *Office Hours uses the Windows System Date (the date set in your Windows operating system), not the NDCMedisoft™ Program Date. For example, if you click the Go to Today button in Office Hours, the calendar will jump to the Windows date and not the NDCMedisoft™ date.*

The Office Hours schedule, shown in the right half of the screen, is a listing of time slots for a particular day for a specific provider. The provider's name and number are displayed at the top to the right of the shortcut buttons. The provider can be easily changed by clicking the triangle button in the Provider box.

Program Options

When Office Hours is installed in a medical practice, it is set up to reflect the needs of that particular practice. Most offices that use NDCMedisoft™

already have Office Hours set up and running. However, if NDCMedisoft™ is just being installed, the options to set up the Office Hours program can be found in the Program Options dialog box, which is accessed by clicking Program Options on the Office Hours File menu.

Entering and Exiting Office Hours

Office Hours can be started from within NDCMedisoft™ or directly from Windows. To access Office Hours from within NDCMedisoft™, click Appointment Book on the Activities menu. Office Hours can also be started by clicking the corresponding shortcut button on the toolbar.

To start Office Hours without entering NDCMedisoft™ first:

1. Click the Start button on the Windows task bar.

2. Click NDCMedisoft™ on the Programs submenu.

3. Click Office Hours on the NDCMedisoft™ submenu.

The Office Hours program is closed by clicking Exit on the Office Hours File menu, or by clicking the Exit button on its toolbar. If Office Hours was started from within NDCMedisoft™, exiting will return you to NDCMedisoft™. If Office Hours was started directly from Windows, clicking Exit will return you to the Windows desktop.

Entering Appointments

Entering an appointment begins with selecting the provider for whom the appointment is being scheduled. The current provider is listed in the Provider box at the top right of the screen. Clicking the triangle button displays a drop-down list of providers in the system. To choose a different provider, click the name of the provider on the drop-down list.

After the provider is selected, the date of the desired appointment must be chosen. Dates are changed by clicking the Day, Week, Month, and Year right and left arrow buttons located under the calendar. After the provider and date have been selected, patient appointments can be entered.

Appointments are entered by clicking the Appointment Entry shortcut button or by double-clicking in a time slot on the schedule. When either of those actions is taken, the New Appointment Entry dialog box is displayed (see Figure A-2 on page 144). The dialog box contains the following fields:

Chart A patient's chart number is chosen from the Chart drop-down list. To select the desired patient, click on the name and press Enter. If you are setting up an appointment for a new patient who has not been assigned a chart number, skip this box and key the patient's name in the Name box.

Name Once a patient's chart is selected from the Chart drop-down list, NDCMedisoft™ displays the patient's name in the Name box. If a patient does not have a chart number, key the patient's name in this box.

Phone After selecting a patient's chart, that patient's phone number is automatically entered in the Phone box.

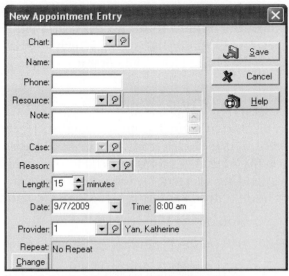

Figure A-2   New Appointment Entry Dialog Box

Resource This box is used if the practice assigns codes to resources, such as exam rooms or equipment.

Note Any special information about an appointment is entered in the Note box.

Case The case that pertains to the appointment is selected from the drop-down list of cases.

Reason Reason codes can be set up in the program to reflect the reason for an appointment.

Length The amount of time an appointment will take (in minutes) is entered in the Length box by keying the number of minutes or by using the up and down arrows.

Date The Date box displays the date that is currently displayed on the calendar. If this is not the desired date, it may be changed by keying in a different date or by clicking the triangle button and using the pop-up calendar that appears.

Time The Time box displays the appointment time that is currently selected on the schedule. If this is not the desired time, it may be changed by keying in a different time.

Provider The provider who will be treating the patient during this appointment is selected from the drop-down list of providers.

Repeat The Repeat box is used to enter appointments that recur on a regular basis.

 After the boxes in the New Appointment Entry dialog box have been completed, clicking the Save button enters the information on the schedule. The patient's name appears in the time slot corresponding to the appoint-

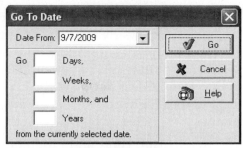

Figure A-3 *Go To Date Dialog Box*

ment time. In addition, information about the appointment appears in the lower left corner of the Office Hours window.

Looking for a Future Date

Often a patient will need a follow-up appointment at a certain time in the future. For example, suppose a physician has seen a certain patient on a particular day and would like a checkup appointment in three weeks. The most efficient way to search for a future appointment in Office Hours is to use the Go to a Date shortcut button on the toolbar. (This feature can also be accessed on the Edit menu.)

Clicking the Go to a Date shortcut button displays the Go to Date dialog box (see Figure A-3). Within the dialog box, the Date From box indicates the current date in the appointment search. Four other boxes offer options for locating a date a specific number of days, weeks, months, or years in the future from the date indicated in the Date From box. After a number is entered in one of the four boxes, clicking the Go button closes the dialog box and begins the search. The system locates the future date and displays the calendar schedule for that date.

Computer Exercise A-1

Enter an appointment for Herbert Bell at 2:30 P.M. on Monday, September 7, 2009. The appointment is 15 minutes in length and is with Dr. Katherine Yan.

1. Start NDCMedisoft™. Start Office Hours by clicking the Appointment Book shortcut button on the toolbar.

2. Verify that "1- Yan, Katherine" is displayed in the Provider box.

3. Change the date on the calendar to Monday, September 7, 2009. Use the forward arrow keys to change the month and year, and then click the day in the calendar itself.

4. In the schedule, under Column 1, double-click the 2:30 P.M. time slot. (You may need to use the scroll bar to view 2:30 P.M.) The New Appointment Entry dialog box is displayed.

5. Click Herbert Bell from the list of names on the drop-down list in the Chart box and press Enter. The system automatically fills in a number of boxes in the dialog box, such as the patient's name and phone number.

6. Accept the default entry in the Case box.

7. Notice that the Length box already contains an entry of 15 minutes. This is the default appointment length set up in NDCMedisoft™. Since Herbert Bell's appointment is for an annual exam, this entry must be changed to 60 minutes. Key *60* in the Length box or use the up arrow next to the length box to change the appointment length to 60 minutes.

8. Verify the entries in the Date, Time, and Provider boxes and then click the Save button. NDCMedisoft™ saves the appointment, closes the dialog box, and displays the appointment on the schedule, as well as in the lower left corner of the Office Hours window. Herbert Bell's name is displayed in the 2:30 P.M. time slot on the schedule.

Computer Exercise A-2

Enter the following appointments with Dr. Katherine Yan.

1. The first appointment is Monday (September 7, 2009) at 3:30 P.M. for John Fitzwilliams, 30 minutes in length. Verify that "1-Yan, Katherine" is displayed in the Provider box.

2. In the schedule, double-click the 3:30 P.M. time-slot box.

3. Select John Fitzwilliams on the Chart drop-down list.

4. Press the Enter key. The program automatically completes several boxes in the dialog box.

5. Press the Tab key until the entry in the Length box is highlighted.

6. Key *30* in the Length box or click the up arrow once to change the length to 30 minutes.

7. Click the Save button. Verify that the appointment for John Fitzwilliams appears on the schedule for September 7, 2009, at 3:30 P.M. for a length of 30 minutes.

8. Enter an appointment on Monday, September 7, 2009, at 4:00 P.M. for Leila Patterson, 15 minutes in length.

9. Enter an appointment on Tuesday, September 8, 2009, at 1:30 P.M. for James Smith, 30 minutes in length.

10. Schedule an appointment two weeks after September 8, 2009, for James Smith at 12:15 P.M., 15 minutes in length. Click the Go To a Date shortcut button.

11. Key 2 in the Go __ Weeks box. Click the Go button. The program closes the Go To Date box and displays the appointment on the schedule for September 22, 2009.

12. Enter James Smith's appointment.

Computer Exercise A-3

Enter these appointments with Dr. Katherine Yan.

1. Verify that Dr. Katherine Yan is selected in the Provider drop-down box.

2. Enter an appointment for Tuesday, September 29, 2009, at 1:30 P.M. for Janine Bell, 15 minutes in length.

3. Use Office Hours' Go to a Date feature to schedule an appointment three weeks from September 29, 2009, at 2:30 P.M. for Sarina Bell, 30 minutes in length.

Searching for Available Appointment Time

Often it is necessary to search for available appointment space on a particular day of the week and at a specific time. For example, a patient needs a 30-minute appointment and would like it to be during his lunch hour, which is from 12:00 P.M. to 1:00 P.M. He can get away from the office only on Mondays and Fridays. Office Hours makes it easy to locate an appointment slot that meets these requirements with the Search for Open Time Slot shortcut button.

Computer Exercise A-4

Search for the next available appointment slot beginning September 8, 2009, with Dr. Yan, on a Thursday or Tuesday, between the hours of 1:00 P.M. and 2:30 P.M.

1. Change the Office Hours calendar to September 8, 2009.

2. Verify that Dr. Katherine Yan is displayed next to the Provider box.

3. On the Edit menu, click Find Open Time, or click the Search for Open Time Slot shortcut button. The Find Open Time dialog box is displayed (see Figure A-4).

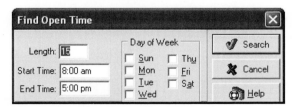

Figure A-4   *Find Open Time Dialog Box*

4. Enter *60* in the Length box. Press the Tab key.

5. Enter *1:00 P.M.* in the Start Time box.

6. Enter *2:30 P.M.* in the End Time box.

7. To search for an appointment on Tuesday or Thursday, click the Tuesday and Thursday boxes in the Day of Week area of the dialog box.

8. Click the Search button to begin looking for an appointment slot. NDCMedisoft™ closes the dialog box and locates the first available time slot that meets these specifications. The time slot is outlined on the schedule.

9. Double-click the selected time slot. Click Maritza Ramos on the drop-down list in the Name box.

10. Press the Tab key until the cursor is in the Length box.

11. Key *60* and press the Tab key.

12. Click the Save button.

13. Verify that the appointment has been entered by looking at the schedule.

Entering Appointments for New Patients

When a new patient phones the office for an appointment, while the prospective patient is still on the phone, most offices obtain basic data and enter it in the appropriate NDCMedisoft™ dialog boxes (Patient/Guarantor and Case). However, if necessary, the appointment can be scheduled in Office Hours before this information is obtained.

Computer Exercise A-5

Schedule Lisa Green, a new patient, for a 45-minute appointment with Dr. Katherine Yan on September 29, 2009, at 1:45 P.M.

1. Go to September 29, 2009 on the schedule and confirm that Dr. Yan is selected as the provider.

2. Double-click the 1:45 P.M. time slot

3. Click in the Name box and key *Green, Lisa.* Press the Tab key to move the cursor to the Phone box.

4. Key *6145553604* in the Phone box and press Tab four times.

5. Key *45* in the Length box.

6. Click the Save button. Check to see that the appointment is displayed on the September 29, 2009 schedule.

Changing or Deleting Appointments

Very often it is necessary to change a patient's appointment or cancel an appointment. Changing an appointment is accomplished with the Cut and Paste commands on the Office Hours Edit menu.

The following steps are used to reschedule an appointment:

1. Locate the appointment that needs to be changed. Make sure the appointment slot is visible on the schedule.

2. Click on the existing time-slot box. A black border surrounds the slot to indicate that it is selected.

3. Click Cut on the Edit menu. The appointment disappears from the schedule.

4. Click the date on the calendar when the appointment is to be rescheduled.

5. Click the desired time-slot box on the schedule. The slot becomes active.

6. Click Paste on the Edit menu. The patient's name appears in the new time-slot box.

The following steps are used to cancel an appointment without rescheduling:

1. Locate the appointment on the schedule.

2. Click the time-slot box to select the appointment.

3. Click Cut on the Edit menu. The appointment disappears from the schedule.

Computer Exercise A-6

Reschedule Janine Bell's appointment.

1. Verify that Dr. Yan is selected as the Provider in Office Hours.

2. Go to Tuesday, September 29, 2009, on the calendar.

3. Locate Janine Bell's 1:30 P.M. appointment on the schedule. Click the 1:30 P.M. time-slot box.

4. Click Cut on the Edit menu. Janine Bell's appointment is removed from the 1:30 P.M. time-slot box. (You may also use the right mouse click shortcut.)

5. Go to Thursday, October 1, 2009, and click the 3:00 P.M. time-slot box.

6. Click Paste on the Edit menu. Janine Bell's name is displayed in the 3:00 P.M. time-slot box for October 1, 2009.

Previewing and Printing Schedules

In most medical offices, providers' schedules are printed on a daily basis. To view a list of all appointments for a provider for a given day, click Appointment List from the Office Hours Reports menu. The report can be previewed on-screen or sent directly to the printer. If the preview option is selected, the appointment list is displayed in a preview window (see Figure A-5 on page 150). Various buttons are used to view the schedule at different sizes, to move from page to page, to print the schedule, and to save the schedule as a file. Clicking the Close button closes the preview window.

The schedule can also be printed by clicking the Print Appointment List shortcut button, without using the Preview option. (Office Hours prints the schedule for the provider who is listed in the Provider box. To print the schedule of a different provider, change the entry in the Provider box before printing the schedule.)

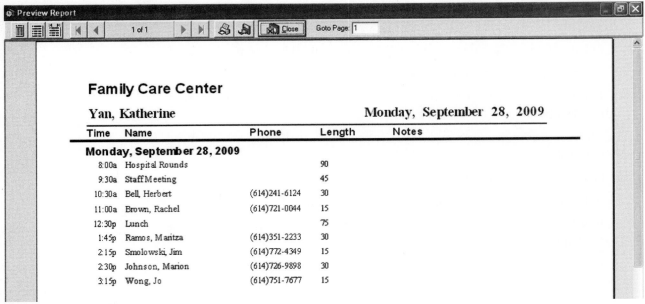

Figure A-5 *Preview Report Dialog Box*

Computer Exercise A-7

Print Dr. Katherine Yan's schedule for September 7, 2009.

1. Confirm that Dr. Katherine Yan is selected as the provider.

2. Go to Monday, September 7, 2009, on the calendar.

3. Click Appointment List on the Office Hours Reports menu. The Report Setup dialog box appears.

4. Under Print Selection, click the button that sends the report directly to the printer, and then click the Start button.

5. The Data Selection dialog box appears. Enter September 7, 2009, in both date boxes.

6. In both provider boxes, select 1 for Dr. Yan. Then click the OK button.

7. The Print dialog box appears. Click OK to print the report.

8. Close the Office Hours program, and then exit NDCMedisoft™.

9. Make a backup copy of your work on exiting. Label the file *PBApp.mbk.*

Source Documents

PATIENT INFORMATION FORM

THIS SECTION REFERS TO PATIENT ONLY

Name: Juan Lomos	Sex: M	Marital Status: ☐ S ☒ M ☐ D ☐ W	Birth Date: 7/21/52

Address: 12 Briar Lane		SS#: 716-83-0061

City: Stephenson	State: OH	Zip: 60089	Employer: Stephenson Wire Works (full-time)

Home Phone: 614-221-0202	Employer's Address: 125 Stephenson Road

Work Phone: 614-525-0215	City: Stephenson	State: OH	Zip: 60089

Spouse's Name:	Spouse's Employer:

Emergency Contact:	Relationship:	Phone #:

FILL IN IF PATIENT IS A MINOR

Parent/Guardian's Name:	Sex:	Marital Status: ☐ S ☐ M ☐ D ☐ W	Birth Date:

Phone:	SS#:

Address:	Employer:

City:	State:	Zip:	Employer's Address:

Student Status:	City:	State:	Zip:

INSURANCE INFORMATION

Primary Insurance Company: Blue Cross Blue Shield	Secondary Insurance Company:

Subscriber's Name: Juan Lomos	Birth Date: 7/21/52	Subscriber's Name:	Birth Date:

Plan: Traditional	SS#: 716-83-0061	Plan:

Policy #: 716830061	Group #: 126	Policy #:	Group #:

Copayment/Deductible: $250	Price Code: A

OTHER INFORMATION

Reason for visit: Auto accident--back injury	Allergy to Medication (list):

Name of referring physician:	If auto accident, list date and state in which it occurred: OH -- 8/8/09

Regardless of any insurance coverage I may or may not have, it is my responsibility to pay the entire bill. In the event that this office needs to obtain legal assistance in collection of any unpaid balance, I agree to pay costs and attorney fees, as allowable by law. I authorize the release of the above patient's medical records for billing purposes. I authorize payment of medical benefits to Dr. Katherine Yan, Dr. Jessica Rudner, or Dr. John Rudner.

Juan Lomos	9/4/09
(Patient's Signature/Parent or Guardian's Signature)	(Date)

Family Care Center
285 Stephenson Boulevard
Stephenson, OH 60089
614-555-0100

From the Desk of Dr. Katherine Yan

Date   9/4/2009
_____

Patient   Juan Lomos
_____

Physician's Notes
_____
Condition related to automobile accident in Ohio on 8/8/09
_____

_____
Patient was hospitalized from 8/8/09 to 8/14/09
_____
Patient was partially disabled from 8/8/09 to 8/19/09
_____

_____
Patient remained partially disabled from 8/20/09 to 9/1/09.
_____

PATIENT INFORMATION FORM

THIS SECTION REFERS TO PATIENT ONLY

Name: Cedera Lomos	Sex: F	Marital Status: ☐ S ☒ M ☐ D ☐ W	Birth Date: 5/21/57

Address: 12 Briar Lane	SS#: 717-87-0054

City: Stephenson	State: OH	Zip: 60089	Employer: The Oyster Bar (full-time)

Home Phone: 614-221-0202	Employer's Address:

Work Phone: 614-299-0313	City: Stephenson	State: OH	Zip: 60089

Spouse's Name:	Spouse's Employer:

Emergency Contact:	Relationship:	Phone #:

FILL IN IF PATIENT IS A MINOR

Parent/Guardian's Name:	Sex:	Marital Status: ☐ S ☐ M ☐ D ☐ W	Birth Date:

Phone:	SS#:

Address:	Employer:

City:	State:	Zip:	Employer's Address:

Student Status:	City:	State:	Zip:

INSURANCE INFORMATION

Primary Insurance Company: Blue Cross/Blue Shield	Secondary Insurance Company: Physician's Alliance of Ohio

Subscriber's Name: Juan Lomos	Birth Date: 7/21/52	Rel. to Insured spouse	Subscriber's Name: Cedera Lomos	Birth Date: 5/21/57	Rel. to Insured self

Plan: Traditional	SS#: 716-83-0061	Plan: Traditional	SS#: 717-87-0054

Policy #: 716830061	Group #: 126	Policy #: 621382	Group #: A435

Deductible: $250	Price Code: A	Copayment/Deductible: $100	Price Code: A

OTHER INFORMATION

Reason for visit: Persistent cough	Allergy to Medication (list): penicillin

Name of referring physician:	If auto accident, list date and state in which it occurred:

Regardless of any insurance coverage I may or may not have, it is my responsibility to pay the entire bill. In the event that this office needs to obtain legal assistance in collection of any unpaid balance, I agree to pay costs and attorney fees, as allowable by law. I authorize the release of the above patient's medical records for billing purposes. I authorize payment of medical benefits to Dr. Katherine Yan, Dr. Jessica Rudner, or Dr. John Rudner.

Cedera Lomos	9/4/09
(Patient's Signature/Parent or Guardian's Signature)	(Date)

PATIENT INFORMATION FORM

THIS SECTION REFERS TO PATIENT ONLY

Name: Lisa Lomos	Sex: F	Marital Status: ☒S ☐M ☐D ☐W	Birth Date: 6/3/04

Address: 12 Briar Lane	SS#: 212-55-3311

City: Stephenson	State: OH	Zip: 60089	Employer:

Home Phone: 614-221-0202	Employer's Address:

Work Phone:	City:	State:	Zip:

Spouse's Name:	Spouse's Employer:

Emergency Contact:	Relationship:	Phone #:

FILL IN IF PATIENT IS A MINOR

Parent/Guardian's Name: Juan Lomos	Sex: M	Marital Status: ☐S ☒M ☐D ☐W	Birth Date: 7/21/52

Phone: 614-221-0202	SS#: 716-83-0061

Address: 12 Briar Lane	Employer: Stephenson Wire Works

City: Stephenson	State: OH	Zip: 60089	Employer's Address: 125 Stephenson Road

Student Status: full-time	City: Stephenson	State: OH	Zip: 60089

INSURANCE INFORMATION

Primary Insurance Company: Blue Cross/Blue Shield	Secondary Insurance Company: Physician's Alliance of Ohio

Subscriber's Name: Juan Lomos	Birth Date: 7/21/52	Rel. to Insured child	Subscriber's Name: Cedera Lomos	Birth Date: 5/21/57	Rel. to Insured child

Plan: Traditional	SS#: 716-83-0061	Plan: Traditional	SS#: 717-87-0054

Policy #: 716830061	Group #: 126	Policy #: 621382	Group #: A435

Deductible: $250	Price Code: A	Copayment/Deductible: $100	Price Code: A

OTHER INFORMATION

Reason for visit: Routine well-child checkup	Allergy to Medication (list):

Name of referring physician:	If auto accident, list date and state in which it occurred:

Regardless of any insurance coverage I may or may not have, it is my responsibility to pay the entire bill. In the event that this office needs to obtain legal assistance in collection of any unpaid balance, I agree to pay costs and attorney fees, as allowable by law. I authorize the release of the above patient's medical records for billing purposes. I authorize payment of medical benefits to Dr. Katherine Yan, Dr. Jessica Rudner, or Dr. John Rudner.

Juan Lomos

(Patient's Signature/Parent or Guardian's Signature)

9/4/09

(Date)

PATIENT INFORMATION FORM

THIS SECTION REFERS TO PATIENT ONLY

Name: Angela Wong	Sex: F	Marital Status: ☒ S ☐ M ☐ D ☐ W	Birth Date: 3/8/92

Address: 10 Maytime Lane, Apt. 3	SS#: 123-62-2111

City: Stephenson	State: OH	Zip: 60089	Employer:

Home Phone: 614-212-0808	Employer's Address:

Work Phone:	City:	State:	Zip:

Spouse's Name:	Spouse's Employer:

Emergency Contact:	Relationship:	Phone #:

FILL IN IF PATIENT IS A MINOR

Parent/Guardian's Name: Peter Wong	Sex: M	Marital Status: ☐ S ☐ M ☒ D ☐ W	Birth Date: 1/17/62

Phone: 614-212-0496	SS#: 419-83-7756

Address: 320 Fourth Street	Employer: U.S. Army (full-time)

City: Stephenson	State: OH	Zip: 60089	Employer's Address: 100 North Andover Road

Student Status: full-time	City: Stephenson	State: OH	Zip: 60089

INSURANCE INFORMATION

Primary Insurance Company: Tricare	Secondary Insurance Company:

Subscriber's Name: Peter Wong	Birth Date: 1/17/62	Rel. to Insured child	Subscriber's Name:	Birth Date:	Rel. to Insured

Plan: Tricare	SS#: 419-83-7756	Plan:	SS#:

Policy #: 397214A	Group #: 647	Policy #:	Group #:

Copayment: $10	Price Code: C	Copayment/Deductible:	Price Code:

OTHER INFORMATION

Reason for visit: Checkup	Allergy to Medication (list):

Name of referring physician:	If auto accident, list date and state in which it occurred:

Regardless of any insurance coverage I may or may not have, it is my responsibility to pay the entire bill. In the event that this office needs to obtain legal assistance in collection of any unpaid balance, I agree to pay costs and attorney fees, as allowable by law. I authorize the release of the above patient's medical records for billing purposes. I authorize payment of medical benefits to Dr. Katherine Yan, Dr. Jessica Rudner, or Dr. John Rudner.

Peter Wong	9/4/09
(Patient's Signature/Parent or Guardian's Signature)	(Date)

Family Care Center
285 Stephenson Boulevard
Stephenson, OH 60089
614-555-0100

Date 9/4/2009

John Fitzwilliams' New Employer

Jenny Designs (full-time)

Family Care Center
285 Stephenson Boulevard
Stephenson, OH 60089
614-555-0100

From the Desk of Dr. Katherine Yan

Date   9/4/2009

Patient   Herbert Mitchell

Physician's Notes

Patient was hospitalized for angina from 8/8/2009 through 9/2/2009.

Medicare representative was contacted and authorized treatment.

Authorization number is 128-33821.

Family Care Center
285 Stephenson Boulevard
Stephenson, OH 60089
614-555-0100

9/4/09
DATE

Cedera Lomos
PATIENT NAME

Dr. Katherine Yan
PROVIDER

LOMCE000
CHART #

OFFICE VISITS - SYMPTOMATIC	
99201	OF--New Patient Minimal
99202	OF--New Patient Low
99203	OF--New Patient Detailed
99204	OF--New Patient Moderate
99205	OF--New Patient High
99211	OF--Established Patient Minimal
99212	OF--Established Patient Low
99213	OF--Established Patient Detailed
99214	OF--Established Patient Moderate
99215	OF--Established Patient High

PREVENTIVE VISITS	
NEW	
99381	Under 1 Year
99382	1 - 4 Years
99383	5 - 11 Years
99384	12 - 17 Years
99385	18 - 39 Years
99386	40 - 64 Years
99387	65 Years & Up
ESTABLISHED	
99391	Under 1 Year
99392	1 - 4 Years
99393	5 - 11 Years
99394	12 - 17 Years
99395	18 - 39 Years
99396	40 - 64 Years
99397	65 Years & Up

PROCEDURES	
12011	Repair of superficial wounds, face
29125	Short arm splint
45378	Colonoscopy--diagnostic
45380	Colonoscopy--biopsy
71010	Chest x-ray, frontal
71020	Chest x-ray, frontal and lateral
73070	Elbow x-ray, AP and lateral

73090	Forearm x-ray, AP and lateral
73100	Wrist x-ray, AP and lateral
73600	Ankle x-ray, AP and lateral
93000	Electrocardiogram--EEG
93015	Treadmill stress test

LABORATORY	
80061	Lipid panel
82270	Hemoccult--stool screening
82465	Cholesterol test
82947	Glucose--quantitative
82951	Glucose tolerance test
83718	HDL cholesterol test
85007	Manual WBC
85025	CBC w/diff.
85651	Erythrocyte sed rate--ESR
86585	Tine test
87040	Strep culture
87430	Strep screen
87086	Urine colony count
87088	Urine culture

INJECTIONS	
90471	Immunization administration
90657	Influenza injection, under 35 months
90658	Influenza injection, older than 3 years
90703	Tetanus immunization
90707	MMR immunization

REFERRING PHYSICIAN

NPI

NOTES

AUTHORIZATION #

DIAGNOSIS

473.9

PAYMENT AMOUNT

9/4/09
DATE

Family Care Center
285 Stephenson Boulevard
Stephenson, OH 60089
614-555-0100

Dr. Katherine Yan
PROVIDER

Lisa Lomos
PATIENT NAME

LOMLI000
CHART #

OFFICE VISITS - SYMPTOMATIC	
99201	OF--New Patient Minimal
99202	OF--New Patient Low
99203	OF--New Patient Detailed
99204	OF--New Patient Moderate
99205	OF--New Patient High
99211	OF--Established Patient Minimal
99212	OF--Established Patient Low
99213	OF--Established Patient Detailed
99214	OF--Established Patient Moderate
99215	OF--Established Patient High
PREVENTIVE VISITS	
NEW	
99381	Under 1 Year
99382	1 - 4 Years
99383	5 - 11 Years
99384	12 - 17 Years
99385	18 - 39 Years
99386	40 - 64 Years
99387	65 Years & Up
ESTABLISHED	
99391	Under 1 Year
99392	1 - 4 Years
99393	5 - 11 Years
99394	12 - 17 Years
99395	18 - 39 Years
99396	40 - 64 Years
99397	65 Years & Up
PROCEDURES	
12011	Repair of superficial wounds, face
29125	Short arm splint
45378	Colonoscopy--diagnostic
45380	Colonoscopy--biopsy
71010	Chest x-ray, frontal
71020	Chest x-ray, frontal and lateral
73070	Elbow x-ray, AP and lateral

73090	Forearm x-ray, AP and lateral
73100	Wrist x-ray, AP and lateral
73600	Ankle x-ray, AP and lateral
93000	Electrocardiogram--EEG
93015	Treadmill stress test
LABORATORY	
80061	Lipid panel
82270	Hemoccult--stool screening
82465	Cholesterol test
82947	Glucose--quantitative
82951	Glucose tolerance test
83718	HDL cholesterol test
85007	Manual WBC
85025	CBC w/diff.
85651	Erythrocyte sed rate--ESR
86585	Tine test
87040	Strep culture
87430	Strep screen
87086	Urine colony count
87088	Urine culture
INJECTIONS	
90471	Immunization administration
90657	Influenza injection, under 35 months
90658	Influenza injection, older than 3 years
90703	Tetanus immunization
90707	MMR immunization

REFERRING PHYSICIAN

NPI

NOTES

AUTHORIZATION #

DIAGNOSIS
v20.2, v06.4

PAYMENT AMOUNT

Family Care Center
285 Stephenson Boulevard
Stephenson, OH 60089
614-555-0100

9/4/09
DATE

Leila Patterson
PATIENT NAME

Dr. Katherine Yan
PROVIDER

PATLE000
CHART #

OFFICE VISITS - SYMPTOMATIC	
99201	OF--New Patient Minimal
99202	OF--New Patient Low
99203	OF--New Patient Detailed
99204	OF--New Patient Moderate
99205	OF--New Patient High
99211	OF--Established Patient Minimal
99212	OF--Established Patient Low
99213	OF--Established Patient Detailed
99214	OF--Established Patient Moderate
99215	OF--Established Patient High

PREVENTIVE VISITS	

NEW	
99381	Under 1 Year
99382	1 - 4 Years
99383	5 - 11 Years
99384	12 - 17 Years
99385	18 - 39 Years
99386	40 - 64 Years
99387	65 Years & Up

ESTABLISHED	
99391	Under 1 Year
99392	1 - 4 Years
99393	5 - 11 Years
99394	12 - 17 Years
99395	18 - 39 Years
99396	40 - 64 Years
99397	65 Years & Up

PROCEDURES	
12011	Repair of superficial wounds, face
29125	Short arm splint
45378	Colonoscopy--diagnostic
45380	Colonoscopy--biopsy
71010	Chest x-ray, frontal
71020	Chest x-ray, frontal and lateral
73070	Elbow x-ray, AP and lateral

73090	Forearm x-ray, AP and lateral
73100	Wrist x-ray, AP and lateral
73600	Ankle x-ray, AP and lateral
93000	Electrocardiogram--EEG
93015	Treadmill stress test

LABORATORY	
80061	Lipid panel
82270	Hemoccult--stool screening
82465	Cholesterol test
82947	Glucose--quantitative
82951	Glucose tolerance test
83718	HDL cholesterol test
85007	Manual WBC
85025	CBC w/diff.
85651	Erythrocyte sed rate--ESR
86585	Tine test
87040	Strep culture
87430	Strep screen
87086	Urine colony count
87088	Urine culture

INJECTIONS	
90471	Immunization administration
90657	Influenza injection, under 35 months
90658	Influenza injection, older than 3 years
90703	Tetanus immunization
90707	MMR immunization

REFERRING PHYSICIAN

NPI

NOTES

AUTHORIZATION #

DIAGNOSIS
272.0

PAYMENT AMOUNT

PATIENT INFORMATION FORM

THIS SECTION REFERS TO PATIENT ONLY

Name: Leila Patterson		Sex: F	Marital Status: ☒S ☐M ☐D ☐W	Birth Date: 2/14/49

Address: 2 Woods Street		SS#: 813-32-9549

City: Jefferson	State: OH	Zip: 60093	Employer:

Home Phone: 614-626-2099	Employer's Address:

Work Phone:	City:	State:	Zip:

Spouse's Name:	Spouse's Employer:

Emergency Contact:	Relationship:	Phone #:

FILL IN IF PATIENT IS A MINOR

Parent/Guardian's Name:	Sex:	Marital Status: ☐S ☐M ☐D ☐W	Birth Date:

Phone:	SS#:

Address:	Employer:

City:	State:	Zip:	Employer's Address:

Student Status:	City:	State:	Zip:

INSURANCE INFORMATION

Primary Insurance Company: Oxford	Secondary Insurance Company:

Subscriber's Name: same	Birth Date:	Rel. to Insured self	Subscriber's Name:	Birth Date:	Rel. to Insured

Plan: Traditional	SS#: 813-32-9549	Plan:	SS#:

Policy #: 3042269Y	Group #:	Policy #:	Group #:

Deductible: $500	Price Code: A	Copayment/Deductible:	Price Code:

OTHER INFORMATION

Reason for visit: Cholesterol test	Allergy to Medication (list):

Name of referring physician:	If auto accident, list date and state in which it occurred:

Regardless of any insurance coverage I may or may not have, it is my responsibility to pay the entire bill. In the event that this office needs to obtain legal assistance in collection of any unpaid balance, I agree to pay costs and attorney fees, as allowable by law. I authorize the release of the above patient's medical records for billing purposes. I authorize payment of medical benefits to Dr. Katherine Yan, Dr. Jessica Rudner, or Dr. John Rudner.

Leila Patterson	9/4/09
(Patient's Signature/Parent or Guardian's Signature)	(Date)

Family Care Center
285 Stephenson Boulevard
Stephenson, OH 60089
614-555-0100

New Insurance Carrier: Oxford

Address Tab	PINS Tab
Code: 13	1 Yan, Katherine (PIN): 1234 / Group ID: 5678
Name: Oxford	2 Rudner, John (PIN): 5678 / Group ID: 5678
Street: 100 Colony Ct.	3 Rudner, Jessica (PIN): 9012 / Group ID: 5678
City: Cincinnati	
State: OH	
Zip: 60314	
Phone: 614-555-0014	
Practice ID: 02385496	

Options Tab

Patient Signature on File: Signature on File

Insured Signature on File: Signature on File

Physician Signature on File: Print Name

Print PINs on Forms: PIN Only

Default Billing Method: Electronic

EDI, Codes Tab

EDI Receiver: NDC00

NDC Record Code: 01

Default Payment Application Codes:

Payment: OXFPAY

Adjustment: OXFADJ

Withhold: OXFWIT

Deductible: OXFDED

Take Back: OXFTAK

9/4/09	**Family Care Center**	**Dr. Katherine Yan**
DATE	**285 Stephenson Boulevard**	PROVIDER
	Stephenson, OH 60089	
Ellen Barmenstein	**614-555-0100**	**BAREL000**
PATIENT NAME		CHART #

OFFICE VISITS - SYMPTOMATIC	
99201	OF--New Patient Minimal
99202	OF--New Patient Low
99203	OF--New Patient Detailed
99204	OF--New Patient Moderate
99205	OF--New Patient High
99211	OF--Established Patient Minimal
99212	OF--Established Patient Low
99213	OF--Established Patient Detailed
99214	OF--Established Patient Moderate
99215	OF--Established Patient High
PREVENTIVE VISITS	
NEW	
99381	Under 1 Year
99382	1 - 4 Years
99383	5 - 11 Years
99384	12 - 17 Years
99385	18 - 39 Years
99386	40 - 64 Years
99387	65 Years & Up
ESTABLISHED	
99391	Under 1 Year
99392	1 - 4 Years
99393	5 - 11 Years
99394	12 - 17 Years
99395	18 - 39 Years
99396	40 - 64 Years
99397	65 Years & Up
PROCEDURES	
12011	Repair of superficial wounds, face
29125	Short arm splint
45378	Colonoscopy--diagnostic
45380	Colonoscopy--biopsy
71010	Chest x-ray, frontal
71020	Chest x-ray, frontal and lateral
73070	Elbow x-ray, AP and lateral

73090	Forearm x-ray, AP and lateral
73100	Wrist x-ray, AP and lateral
73600	Ankle x-ray, AP and lateral
93000	Electrocardiogram--EEG
93015	Treadmill stress test
LABORATORY	
80061	Lipid panel
82270	Hemoccult--stool screening
82465	Cholesterol test
82947	Glucose--quantitative
82951	Glucose tolerance test
83718	HDL cholesterol test
85007	Manual WBC
85025	CBC w/diff.
85651	Erythrocyte sed rate--ESR
86585	Tine test
87040	Strep culture
87430	Strep screen
87086	Urine colony count
87088	Urine culture
INJECTIONS	
90471	Immunization administration
90657	Influenza injection, under 35 months
90658	Influenza injection, older than 3 years
90703	Tetanus immunization
90707	MMR immunization

REFERRING PHYSICIAN	NPI	NOTES
AUTHORIZATION #		
DIAGNOSIS		
v04.81		
PAYMENT AMOUNT		

Family Care Center
285 Stephenson Boulevard
Stephenson, OH 60089
614-555-0100

9/4/09
DATE

Hiro Tanaka
PATIENT NAME

Dr. Katherine Yan
PROVIDER

TANHI000
CHART #

OFFICE VISITS - SYMPTOMATIC	
99201	OF--New Patient Minimal
99202	OF--New Patient Low
99203	OF--New Patient Detailed
99204	OF--New Patient Moderate
99205	OF--New Patient High
99211	OF--Established Patient Minimal
99212	OF--Established Patient Low
99213	OF--Established Patient Detailed
99214	OF--Established Patient Moderate
99215	OF--Established Patient High
PREVENTIVE VISITS	
NEW	
99381	Under 1 Year
99382	1 - 4 Years
99383	5 - 11 Years
99384	12 - 17 Years
99385	18 - 39 Years
99386	40 - 64 Years
99387	65 Years & Up
ESTABLISHED	
99391	Under 1 Year
99392	1 - 4 Years
99393	5 - 11 Years
99394	12 - 17 Years
99395	18 - 39 Years
99396	40 - 64 Years
99397	65 Years & Up
PROCEDURES	
12011	Repair of superficial wounds, face
29125	Short arm splint
45378	Colonoscopy--diagnostic
45380	Colonoscopy--biopsy
71010	Chest x-ray, frontal
71020	Chest x-ray, frontal and lateral
73070	Elbow x-ray, AP and lateral

73090	Forearm x-ray, AP and lateral
73100	Wrist x-ray, AP and lateral
73600	Ankle x-ray, AP and lateral
93000	Electrocardiogram--EEG
93015	Treadmill stress test
LABORATORY	
80061	Lipid panel
82270	Hemoccult--stool screening
82465	Cholesterol test
82947	Glucose--quantitative
82951	Glucose tolerance test
83718	HDL cholesterol test
85007	Manual WBC
85025	CBC w/diff.
85651	Erythrocyte sed rate--ESR
86585	Tine test
87040	Strep culture
87430	Strep screen
87086	Urine colony count
87088	Urine culture
INJECTIONS	
90471	Immunization administration
90657	Influenza injection, under 35 months
90658	Influenza injection, older than 3 years
90703	Tetanus immunization
90707	MMR immunization

REFERRING PHYSICIAN   NPI

AUTHORIZATION #

DIAGNOSIS
848.9

PAYMENT AMOUNT
$10 copayment, check #3022

NOTES

9/4/09
DATE

Elizabeth Jones
PATIENT NAME

Family Care Center
285 Stephenson Boulevard
Stephenson, OH 60089
614-555-0100

Dr. Katherine Yan
PROVIDER

JONEL000
CHART #

	OFFICE VISITS - SYMPTOMATIC
99201	OF--New Patient Minimal
99202	OF--New Patient Low
99203	OF--New Patient Detailed
99204	OF--New Patient Moderate
99205	OF--New Patient High
99211	OF--Established Patient Minimal
99212	OF--Established Patient Low
99213	OF--Established Patient Detailed
99214	OF--Established Patient Moderate
99215	OF--Established Patient High
	PREVENTIVE VISITS
	NEW
99381	Under 1 Year
99382	1 - 4 Years
99383	5 - 11 Years
99384	12 - 17 Years
99385	18 - 39 Years
99386	40 - 64 Years
99387	65 Years & Up
	ESTABLISHED
99391	Under 1 Year
99392	1 - 4 Years
99393	5 - 11 Years
99394	12 - 17 Years
99395	18 - 39 Years
99396	40 - 64 Years
99397	65 Years & Up
	PROCEDURES
12011	Repair of superficial wounds, face
29125	Short arm splint
45378	Colonoscopy--diagnostic
45380	Colonoscopy--biopsy
71010	Chest x-ray, frontal
71020	Chest x-ray, frontal and lateral
73070	Elbow x-ray, AP and lateral

73090	Forearm x-ray, AP and lateral
73100	Wrist x-ray, AP and lateral
73600	Ankle x-ray, AP and lateral
93000	Electrocardiogram--EEG
93015	Treadmill stress test
	LABORATORY
80061	Lipid panel
82270	Hemoccult--stool screening
82465	Cholesterol test
82947	Glucose--quantitative
82951	Glucose tolerance test
83718	HDL cholesterol test
85007	Manual WBC
85025	CBC w/diff.
85651	Erythrocyte sed rate--ESR
86585	Tine test
87040	Strep culture
87430	Strep screen
87086	Urine colony count
87088	Urine culture
	INJECTIONS
90471	Immunization administration
90657	Influenza injection, under 35 months
90658	Influenza injection, older than 3 years
90703	Tetanus immunization
90707	MMR immunization

REFERRING PHYSICIAN

NPI

NOTES

AUTHORIZATION #

DIAGNOSIS
461.9

PAYMENT AMOUNT
$15 copayment, check #609

Family Care Center
285 Stephenson Boulevard
Stephenson, OH 60089
614-555-0100

9/4/09
DATE

Sarina Bell
PATIENT NAME

Dr. Katherine Yan
PROVIDER

BELSA001
CHART #

	OFFICE VISITS - SYMPTOMATIC
99201	OF--New Patient Minimal
99202	OF--New Patient Low
99203	OF--New Patient Detailed
99204	OF--New Patient Moderate
99205	OF--New Patient High
99211	OF--Established Patient Minimal
99212	OF--Established Patient Low
99213	OF--Established Patient Detailed
99214	OF--Established Patient Moderate
99215	OF--Established Patient High

	PREVENTIVE VISITS
	NEW
99381	Under 1 Year
99382	1 - 4 Years
99383	5 - 11 Years
99384	12 - 17 Years
99385	18 - 39 Years
99386	40 - 64 Years
99387	65 Years & Up
	ESTABLISHED
99391	Under 1 Year
99392	1 - 4 Years
99393	5 - 11 Years
99394	12 - 17 Years
99395	18 - 39 Years
99396	40 - 64 Years
99397	65 Years & Up

	PROCEDURES
12011	Repair of superficial wounds, face
29125	Short arm splint
45378	Colonoscopy--diagnostic
45380	Colonoscopy--biopsy
71010	Chest x-ray, frontal
71020	Chest x-ray, frontal and lateral
73070	Elbow x-ray, AP and lateral

73090	Forearm x-ray, AP and lateral
73100	Wrist x-ray, AP and lateral
73600	Ankle x-ray, AP and lateral
93000	Electrocardiogram--EEG
93015	Treadmill stress test

	LABORATORY
80061	Lipid panel
82270	Hemoccult--stool screening
82465	Cholesterol test
82947	Glucose--quantitative
82951	Glucose tolerance test
83718	HDL cholesterol test
85007	Manual WBC
85025	CBC w/diff.
85651	Erythrocyte sed rate--ESR
86585	Tine test
87040	Strep culture
87430	Strep screen
87086	Urine colony count
87088	Urine culture

	INJECTIONS
90471	Immunization administration
90657	Influenza injection, under 35 months
90658	Influenza injection, older than 3 years
90703	Tetanus immunization
90707	MMR immunization

REFERRING PHYSICIAN

NPI

NOTES

AUTHORIZATION #

DIAGNOSIS
034.0

PAYMENT AMOUNT
$15 copayment, check #309

BLUE CROSS BLUE SHIELD
340 Preston Boulevard
Columbus, OH 60220

PROVIDER REMITTANCE
THIS IS NOT A BILL
A PAYMENT SUMMARY AND AN EXPLANATION OF
CODES ARE AT THE END OF THIS STATEMENT

FAMILY CARE CENTER
285 STEPHENSON BLVD.
STEPHENSON, OH 60089

PAGE:	1 OF 1
DATE:	9/2/09
ID NUMBER:	36094251

PROVIDER: KATHERINE YAN, M.D.

PATIENT: FELDMAN STANLEY

PROC CODE	FROM DATE	THRU DATE	TREAT -MENT	STATUS CODE	AMOUNT CHRGD	AMOUNT ALLWD	COPAY/ DEDUCT	AMOUNT APPRVD	PATIENT BALANCE
93015	7/28/09	7/28/09	1	A	325.00	325.00	.00	260.00	65.00
		TOTALS			325.00	325.00	.00	260.00	65.00

PATIENT: JOHNSON MARION

PROC CODE	FROM DATE	THRU DATE	TREAT -MENT	STATUS CODE	AMOUNT CHRGD	AMOUNT ALLWD	COPAY/ DEDUCT	AMOUNT APPRVD	PATIENT BALANCE
99215	7/15/09	7/15/09	1	A	135.00	135.00	.00	108.00	27.00
93000	7/15/09	7/15/09	1	A	70.00	70.00	.00	56.00	14.00
71010	7/15/09	7/15/09	1	A	80.00	80.00	.00	64.00	16.00
82947	8/18/09	8/18/09	1	A	21.00	21.00	.00	16.80	4.20
		TOTALS			306.00	306.00	.00	244.80	61.20

PATIENT: SMITH JAMES

PROC CODE	FROM DATE	THRU DATE	TREAT -MENT	STATUS CODE	AMOUNT CHRGD	AMOUNT ALLWD	COPAY/ DEDUCT	AMOUNT APPRVD	PATIENT BALANCE
99212	7/8/09	7/8/09	1	A	44.00	44.00	.00	35.20	8.80
99212	8/17/09	8/17/09	1	A	44.00	44.00	.00	35.20	8.80
		TOTALS			88.00	88.00	.00	70.40	17.60

PAYMENT SUMMARY		TOTAL ALL CLAIMS		EFT INFORMATION	
TOTAL AMOUNT PAID	575.20	AMOUNT CHARGES	719.00	NUMBER	36094251
PRIOR CREDIT BALANCE	.00	AMOUNT ALLOWED	719.00	DATE	9/2/09
CURRENT CREDIT DEFERRED	.00	DEDUCTIBLE	.00	AMOUNT	575.20
PRIOR CREDIT APPLIED	.00	COPAY	.00		
NEW CREDIT BALANCE	.00	OTHER REDUCTION	.00		
NET DISBURSED	575.20	AMOUNT APPROVED	575.20		

STATUS CODES:
A - APPROVED   AJ - ADJUSTMENT   IP - IN PROCESS   R - REJECTED   V - VOID

BLUE CROSS BLUE SHIELD
340 Preston Boulevard
Columbus, OH 60220

PROVIDER REMITTANCE
THIS IS NOT A BILL
A PAYMENT SUMMARY AND AN EXPLANATION OF
CODES ARE AT THE END OF THIS STATEMENT

FAMILY CARE CENTER
285 STEPHENSON BLVD.
STEPHENSON, OH 60089

PAGE: 1 OF 1
DATE: 9/7/09
ID NUMBER: 3574896

PROVIDER: KATHERINE YAN, M.D.

PATIENT: BARMENSTEIN ELLEN

PROC CODE	FROM DATE	THRU DATE	TREAT -MENT	STATUS CODE	AMOUNT CHRGD	AMOUNT ALLWD	COPAY/ DEDUCT	AMOUNT APPRVD	PATIENT BALANCE
99212	8/28/09	8/28/09	1	A	44.00	44.00	.00	35.20	8.80
99211	9/4/09	9/4/09	1	A	30.00	.00	.00	.00	30.00 (See Note A)
90471	9/4/09	9/4/09	1	A	10.00	10.00	.00	8.00	2.00
90658	9/4/09	9/4/09	1	A	12.00	12.00	.00	9.60	2.40
	TOTALS				96.00	66.00	.00	52.80	43.20

A: Not eligible when combined with 90471.

PAYMENT SUMMARY		TOTAL ALL CLAIMS		EFT INFORMATION	
TOTAL AMOUNT PAID	52.80	AMOUNT CHARGES	96.00	NUMBER	3574896
PRIOR CREDIT BALANCE	.00	AMOUNT ALLOWED	66.00	DATE	9/7/09
CURRENT CREDIT DEFERRED	.00	DEDUCTIBLE	.00	AMOUNT	52.80
PRIOR CREDIT APPLIED	.00	COPAY	.00		
NEW CREDIT BALANCE	.00	OTHER REDUCTION	.00		
NET DISBURSED	52.80	AMOUNT APPROVED	52.80		

STATUS CODES:
A - APPROVED   AJ - ADJUSTMENT   IP - IN PROCESS   R - REJECTED   V - VOID

Family Care Center
285 Stephenson Boulevard
Stephenson, OH 60089
614-555-0100

10/30/09
DATE

Janine Bell
PATIENT NAME

Dr. Katherine Yan
PROVIDER

BELJA000
CHART #

OFFICE VISITS - SYMPTOMATIC	
99201	OF--New Patient Minimal
99202	OF--New Patient Low
99203	OF--New Patient Detailed
99204	OF--New Patient Moderate
99205	OF--New Patient High
99211	OF--Established Patient Minimal
99212	OF--Established Patient Low
99213	OF--Established Patient Detailed
99214	OF--Established Patient Moderate
99215	OF--Established Patient High

PREVENTIVE VISITS	
NEW	
99381	Under 1 Year
99382	1 - 4 Years
99383	5 - 11 Years
99384	12 - 17 Years
99385	18 - 39 Years
99386	40 - 64 Years
99387	65 Years & Up
ESTABLISHED	
99391	Under 1 Year
99392	1 - 4 Years
99393	5 - 11 Years
99394	12 - 17 Years
99395	18 - 39 Years
99396	40 - 64 Years
99397	65 Years & Up

PROCEDURES	
12011	Repair of superficial wounds, face
29125	Short arm splint
45378	Colonoscopy--diagnostic
45380	Colonoscopy--biopsy
71010	Chest x-ray, frontal
71020	Chest x-ray, frontal and lateral
73070	Elbow x-ray, AP and lateral

73090	Forearm x-ray, AP and lateral
73100	Wrist x-ray, AP and lateral

PROCEDURES	
73600	Ankle x-ray, AP and lateral
93000	Electrocardiogram--EEG
93015	Treadmill stress test

LABORATORY	
80061	Lipid panel
82270	Hemoccult--stool screening
82465	Cholesterol test
82947	Glucose--quantitative
82951	Glucose tolerance test
83718	HDL cholesterol test
85007	Manual WBC
85025	CBC w/diff.
85651	Erythrocyte sed rate--ESR
86585	Tine test
87040	Strep culture
87430	Strep screen
87086	Urine colony count
87088	Urine culture

INJECTIONS	
90471	Immunization administration
90657	Influenza injection, under 35 months
90658	Influenza injection, older than 3 years
90703	Tetanus immunization
90707	MMR immunization

REFERRING PHYSICIAN

NPI

NOTES

AUTHORIZATION #

DIAGNOSIS
Diabetes mellitus

PAYMENT AMOUNT
$15 copayment, check #33

10/30/09
DATE

Family Care Center
285 Stephenson Boulevard
Stephenson, OH 60089
614-555-0100

Dr. Katherine Yan
PROVIDER

Felix Suarez
PATIENT NAME

SUAFE000
CHART #

OFFICE VISITS - SYMPTOMATIC	
99201	OF--New Patient Minimal
99202	OF--New Patient Low
99203	OF--New Patient Detailed
99204	OF--New Patient Moderate
99205	OF--New Patient High
99211	OF--Established Patient Minimal
99212	OF--Established Patient Low
99213	OF--Established Patient Detailed
99214	OF--Established Patient Moderate
99215	OF--Established Patient High

PREVENTIVE VISITS	
NEW	
99381	Under 1 Year
99382	1 - 4 Years
99383	5 - 11 Years
99384	12 - 17 Years
99385	18 - 39 Years
99386	40 - 64 Years
99387	65 Years & Up
ESTABLISHED	
99391	Under 1 Year
99392	1 - 4 Years
99393	5 - 11 Years
99394	12 - 17 Years
99395	18 - 39 Years
99396	40 - 64 Years
99397	65 Years & Up

PROCEDURES	
12011	Repair of superficial wounds, face
29125	Short arm splint
45378	Colonoscopy--diagnostic
45380	Colonoscopy--biopsy
71010	Chest x-ray, frontal
71020	Chest x-ray, frontal and lateral
73070	Elbow x-ray, AP and lateral

73090	Forearm x-ray, AP and lateral
73100	Wrist x-ray, AP and lateral

PROCEDURES	
73600	Ankle x-ray, AP and lateral
93000	Electrocardiogram--EEG
93015	Treadmill stress test

LABORATORY	
80061	Lipid panel
82270	Hemoccult--stool screening
82465	Cholesterol test
82947	Glucose--quantitative
82951	Glucose tolerance test
83718	HDL cholesterol test
85007	Manual WBC
85025	CBC w/diff.
85651	Erythrocyte sed rate--ESR
86585	Tine test
87040	Strep culture
87430	Strep screen
87086	Urine colony count
87088	Urine culture

INJECTIONS	
90471	Immunization administration
90657	Influenza injection, under 35 months
90658	Influenza injection, older than 3 years
90703	Tetanus immunization
90707	MMR immunization

REFERRING PHYSICIAN

NPI

NOTES

AUTHORIZATION #

DIAGNOSIS
Hemorrhoids

PAYMENT AMOUNT
$15 copayment, check #3011

10/30/09
DATE

Fitzwilliams, Sarah
PATIENT NAME

Family Care Center
285 Stephenson Boulevard
Stephenson, OH 60089
614-555-0100

Dr. Katherine Yan
PROVIDER

FITSA000
CHART #

OFFICE VISITS - SYMPTOMATIC	
99201	OF--New Patient Minimal
99202	OF--New Patient Low
99203	OF--New Patient Detailed
99204	OF--New Patient Moderate
99205	OF--New Patient High
99211	OF--Established Patient Minimal
99212	OF--Established Patient Low
99213	OF--Established Patient Detailed
99214	OF--Established Patient Moderate
99215	OF--Established Patient High
PREVENTIVE VISITS	
NEW	
99381	Under 1 Year
99382	1 - 4 Years
99383	5 - 11 Years
99384	12 - 17 Years
99385	18 - 39 Years
99386	40 - 64 Years
99387	65 Years & Up
ESTABLISHED	
99391	Under 1 Year
99392	1 - 4 Years
99393	5 - 11 Years
99394	12 - 17 Years
99395	18 - 39 Years
99396	40 - 64 Years
99397	65 Years & Up
PROCEDURES	
12011	Repair of superficial wounds, face
29125	Short arm splint
45378	Colonoscopy--diagnostic
45380	Colonoscopy--biopsy
71010	Chest x-ray, frontal
71020	Chest x-ray, frontal and lateral
73070	Elbow x-ray, AP and lateral

73090	Forearm x-ray, AP and lateral
73100	Wrist x-ray, AP and lateral
PROCEDURES	
73600	Ankle x-ray, AP and lateral
93000	Electrocardiogram--EEG
93015	Treadmill stress test
LABORATORY	
80061	Lipid panel
82270	Hemoccult--stool screening
82465	Cholesterol test
82947	Glucose--quantitative
82951	Glucose tolerance test
83718	HDL cholesterol test
85007	Manual WBC
85025	CBC w/diff.
85651	Erythrocyte sed rate--ESR
86585	Tine test
87040	Strep culture
87430	Strep screen
87086	Urine colony count
87088	Urine culture
INJECTIONS	
90471	Immunization administration
90657	Influenza injection, under 35 months
90658	Influenza injection, older than 3 years
90703	Tetanus immunization
90707	MMR immunization

REFERRING PHYSICIAN   NPI

NOTES

AUTHORIZATION #

DIAGNOSIS
Essential hypertension

PAYMENT AMOUNT
$10 copayment, check #345

Family Care Center
285 Stephenson Boulevard
Stephenson, OH 60089
614-555-0100

10/30/09
DATE

Marion Johnson
PATIENT NAME

Dr. Katherine Yan
PROVIDER

JOHMA000
CHART #

OFFICE VISITS - SYMPTOMATIC	
99201	OF--New Patient Minimal
99202	OF--New Patient Low
99203	OF--New Patient Detailed
99204	OF--New Patient Moderate
99205	OF--New Patient High
99211	OF--Established Patient Minimal
99212	OF--Established Patient Low
99213	OF--Established Patient Detailed
99214	OF--Established Patient Moderate
99215	OF--Established Patient High

PREVENTIVE VISITS	
NEW	
99381	Under 1 Year
99382	1 - 4 Years
99383	5 - 11 Years
99384	12 - 17 Years
99385	18 - 39 Years
99386	40 - 64 Years
99387	65 Years & Up
ESTABLISHED	
99391	Under 1 Year
99392	1 - 4 Years
99393	5 - 11 Years
99394	12 - 17 Years
99395	18 - 39 Years
99396	40 - 64 Years
99397	65 Years & Up

PROCEDURES	
12011	Repair of superficial wounds, face
29125	Short arm splint
45378	Colonoscopy--diagnostic
45380	Colonoscopy--biopsy
71010	Chest x-ray, frontal
71020	Chest x-ray, frontal and lateral
73070	Elbow x-ray, AP and lateral

73090	Forearm x-ray, AP and lateral
73100	Wrist x-ray, AP and lateral
73600	Ankle x-ray, AP and lateral
93000	Electrocardiogram--EEG
93015	Treadmill stress test

LABORATORY	
80061	Lipid panel
82270	Hemoccult--stool screening
82465	Cholesterol test
82947	Glucose--quantitative
82951	Glucose tolerance test
83718	HDL cholesterol test
85007	Manual WBC
85025	CBC w/diff.
85651	Erythrocyte sed rate--ESR
86585	Tine test
87040	Strep culture
87430	Strep screen
87086	Urine colony count
87088	Urine culture

INJECTIONS	
90471	Immunization administration
90657	Influenza injection, under 35 months
90658	Influenza injection, older than 3 years
90703	Tetanus immunization
90707	MMR immunization

REFERRING PHYSICIAN

NPI

NOTES

AUTHORIZATION #

DIAGNOSIS
Bronchitis, unqualified

PAYMENT AMOUNT

BLUE CROSS BLUE SHIELD
340 Preston Boulevard
Columbus, OH 60220

PROVIDER REMITTANCE
THIS IS NOT A BILL
A PAYMENT SUMMARY AND AN EXPLANATION OF
CODES ARE AT THE END OF THIS STATEMENT

FAMILY CARE CENTER
285 STEPHENSON BLVD.
STEPHENSON, OH 60089

PAGE: 1 OF 1
DATE: 10/30/09
ID NUMBER: 004567

PROVIDER: KATHERINE YAN, M.D.

PATIENT: LOMOS CEDERA

PROC CODE	FROM DATE	THRU DATE	TREAT -MENT	STATUS CODE	AMOUNT CHRGD	AMOUNT ALLWD	COPAY/ DEDUCT	AMOUNT APPRVD	PATIENT BALANCE
99204	9/4/09	9/4/09	1	A	147.00	147.00	.00	117.60	29.40
		TOTALS			147.00	147.00	.00	117.60	29.40

PATIENT: LOMOS LISA

PROC CODE	FROM DATE	THRU DATE	TREAT -MENT	STATUS CODE	AMOUNT CHRGD	AMOUNT ALLWD	COPAY/ DEDUCT	AMOUNT APPRVD	PATIENT BALANCE
99383	9/4/09	9/4/09	1	A	140.00	140.00	.00	112.00	28.00
90471	9/4/09	9/4/09	1	A	10.00	10.00	.00	8.00	2.00
90707	9/4/09	9/4/09	1	A	105.00	105.00	.00	84.00	21.00
		TOTALS			255.00	255.00	.00	204.00	51.00

PAYMENT SUMMARY		TOTAL ALL CLAIMS		EFT INFORMATION	
TOTAL AMOUNT PAID	321.60	AMOUNT CHARGES	402.00	NUMBER	004567
PRIOR CREDIT BALANCE	.00	AMOUNT ALLOWED	402.00	DATE	10/30/09
CURRENT CREDIT DEFERRED	.00	DEDUCTIBLE	.00	AMOUNT	321.60
PRIOR CREDIT APPLIED	.00	COPAY	.00		
NEW CREDIT BALANCE	.00	OTHER REDUCTION	.00		
NET DISBURSED	321.60	AMOUNT APPROVED	321.60		

STATUS CODES:
A - APPROVED	AJ - ADJUSTMENT	IP - IN PROCESS	R - REJECTED	V - VOID

PATIENT INFORMATION FORM

THIS SECTION REFERS TO PATIENT ONLY

Name: Darla Andrews	Sex: F	Marital Status: ☐ S ☒ M ☐ D ☐ W	Birth Date: 6/8/78

Address: 1 West 8th Street	SS#: 332-49-0432

City: Stephenson	State: OH	Zip: 60089	Employer: Western Drug

Home Phone: 614-241-3321	Employer's Address:

Work Phone: 614-721-0032	City:	State:	Zip:

Spouse's Name:	Spouse's Employer:

Emergency Contact:	Relationship:	Phone #:

FILL IN IF PATIENT IS A MINOR

Parent/Guardian's Name:	Sex:	Marital Status: ☐ S ☐ M ☐ D ☐ W	Birth Date:

Phone:	SS#:

Address:	Employer:

City:	State:	Zip:	Employer's Address:

Student Status:	City:	State:	Zip:

INSURANCE INFORMATION

Primary Insurance Company: Physician's Choice	Secondary Insurance Company:

Subscriber's Name: (same)	Birth Date: 6/8/78	Subscriber's Name:	Birth Date:

Plan:	SS#: 332-49-0432	Plan:

Policy #: 1122191	Group #: 83	Policy #:	Group #:

Copayment: $15	Price Code: B

OTHER INFORMATION

Reason for visit: Chest pain	Allergy to Medication (list):

Name of referring physician:	If auto accident, list date and state in which it occurred:

Regardless of any insurance coverage I may or may not have, it is my responsibility to pay the entire bill. In the event that this office needs to obtain legal assistance in collection of any unpaid balance, I agree to pay costs and attorney fees, as allowable by law. I authorize the release of the above patient's medical records for billing purposes. I authorize payment of medical benefits to Dr. Katherine Yan, Dr. Jessica Rudner, or Dr. John Rudner.

Darla Andrews	11/02/2009
(Patient's Signature/Parent or Guardian's Signature)	(Date)

PATIENT INFORMATION FORM

THIS SECTION REFERS TO PATIENT ONLY

Name: Bill Andrews	Sex: M	Marital Status: ☐ S ☒ M ☐ D ☐ W	Birth Date: 12/1/75

Address:
1 West 8th Street

SS#:
341-59-9392

City: Stephenson	State: OH	Zip: 60089

Employer:
Wheeler, Sampson, Hull (full-time)

Home Phone:
614-241-3321

Employer's Address:

Work Phone:
614-836-8579

City: State: Zip:

Spouse's Name:

Spouse's Employer:

Emergency Contact:

Relationship: Phone #:

FILL IN IF PATIENT IS A MINOR

Parent/Guardian's Name:

Sex:

Marital Status:
☐ S ☐ M ☐ D ☐ W

Birth Date:

Phone:

SS#:

Address:

Employer:

City: State: Zip:

Employer's Address:

Student Status:

City: State: Zip:

INSURANCE INFORMATION

Primary Insurance Company:
Physician's Choice

Secondary Insurance Company:

Subscriber's Name: Darla Andrews	Birth Date: 6/8/78

Subscriber's Name: Birth Date:

Plan:

SS#:
332-49-0432

Plan:

Policy #: 1122191	Group #: 83

Policy #:   Group #:

Copayment $15	Price Code: B

OTHER INFORMATION

Reason for visit:
Routine physical

Allergy to Medication (list):
Penicillin

Name of referring physician:

If auto accident, list date and
state in which it occurred:

Bill Andrews   11/02/2009

(Patient's Signature/Parent or Guardian's Signature)   (Date)

Family Care Center
285 Stephenson Boulevard
Stephenson, OH 60089
614-555-0100

Things to Do Today

Date   **11/2/2009**

Patient   **James Smith**

James Smith has a new address:

100 Meadowlark Lane

Stephenson, OH 60089

Telephone numbers remain the same.

11/2/09
DATE

Darla Andrews
PATIENT NAME

Family Care Center
285 Stephenson Boulevard
Stephenson, OH 60089
614-555-0100

Dr. Katherine Yan
PROVIDER

ANDDA000
CHART #

OFFICE VISITS - SYMPTOMATIC	
99201	OF--New Patient Minimal
99202	OF--New Patient Low
99203	OF--New Patient Detailed
99204	OF--New Patient Moderate
99205	OF--New Patient High
99211	OF--Established Patient Minimal
99212	OF--Established Patient Low
99213	OF--Established Patient Detailed
99214	OF--Established Patient Moderate
99215	OF--Established Patient High
PREVENTIVE VISITS	
NEW	
99381	Under 1 Year
99382	1 - 4 Years
99383	5 - 11 Years
99384	12 - 17 Years
99385	18 - 39 Years
99386	40 - 64 Years
99387	65 Years & Up
ESTABLISHED	
99391	Under 1 Year
99392	1 - 4 Years
99393	5 - 11 Years
99394	12 - 17 Years
99395	18 - 39 Years
99396	40 - 64 Years
99397	65 Years & Up
PROCEDURES	
12011	Repair of superficial wounds, face
29125	Short arm splint
45378	Colonoscopy--diagnostic
45380	Colonoscopy--biopsy
71010	Chest x-ray, frontal
71020	Chest x-ray, frontal and lateral
73070	Elbow x-ray, AP and lateral

73090	Forearm x-ray, AP and lateral
73100	Wrist x-ray, AP and lateral
73600	Ankle x-ray, AP and lateral
93000	Electrocardiogram--EEG
93015	Treadmill stress test
LABORATORY	
80061	Lipid panel
82270	Hemoccult--stool screening
82465	Cholesterol test
82947	Glucose--quantitative
82951	Glucose tolerance test
83718	HDL cholesterol test
85007	Manual WBC
85025	CBC w/diff.
85651	Erythrocyte sed rate--ESR
86585	Tine test
87040	Strep culture
87430	Strep screen
87086	Urine colony count
87088	Urine culture
INJECTIONS	
90471	Immunization administration
90657	Influenza injection, under 35 months
90658	Influenza injection, older than 3 years
90703	Tetanus immunization
90707	MMR immunization

REFERRING PHYSICIAN   NPI

AUTHORIZATION #

DIAGNOSIS
Chest pain

PAYMENT AMOUNT
$15 copayment, check 123

NOTES

11/2/09
DATE

Bill Andrews
PATIENT NAME

Family Care Center
285 Stephenson Boulevard
Stephenson, OH 60089
614-555-0100

Dr. Katherine Yan
PROVIDER

ANDBI000
CHART #

OFFICE VISITS - SYMPTOMATIC	
99201	OF--New Patient Minimal
99202	OF--New Patient Low
99203	OF--New Patient Detailed
99204	OF--New Patient Moderate
99205	OF--New Patient High
99211	OF--Established Patient Minimal
99212	OF--Established Patient Low
99213	OF--Established Patient Detailed
99214	OF--Established Patient Moderate
99215	OF--Established Patient High
PREVENTIVE VISITS	
NEW	
99381	Under 1 Year
99382	1 - 4 Years
99383	5 - 11 Years
99384	12 - 17 Years
99385	18 - 39 Years
99386	40 - 64 Years
99387	65 Years & Up
ESTABLISHED	
99391	Under 1 Year
99392	1 - 4 Years
99393	5 - 11 Years
99394	12 - 17 Years
99395	18 - 39 Years
99396	40 - 64 Years
99397	65 Years & Up
PROCEDURES	
12011	Repair of superficial wounds, face
29125	Short arm splint
45378	Colonoscopy--diagnostic
45380	Colonoscopy--biopsy
71010	Chest x-ray, frontal
71020	Chest x-ray, frontal and lateral
73070	Elbow x-ray, AP and lateral

73090	Forearm x-ray, AP and lateral
73100	Wrist x-ray, AP and lateral
73600	Ankle x-ray, AP and lateral
93000	Electrocardiogram--EEG
93015	Treadmill stress test
LABORATORY	
80061	Lipid panel
82270	Hemoccult--stool screening
82465	Cholesterol test
82947	Glucose--quantitative
82951	Glucose tolerance test
83718	HDL cholesterol test
85007	Manual WBC
85025	CBC w/diff.
85651	Erythrocyte sed rate--ESR
86585	Tine test
87040	Strep culture
87430	Strep screen
87086	Urine colony count
87088	Urine culture
INJECTIONS	
90471	Immunization administration
90657	Influenza injection, under 35 months
90658	Influenza injection, older than 3 years
90703	Tetanus immunization
90707	MMR immunization

REFERRING PHYSICIAN

NPI

NOTES

AUTHORIZATION #

DIAGNOSIS
Preventive physical exam

PAYMENT AMOUNT
$15 copayment, check 124

Family Care Center
285 Stephenson Boulevard
Stephenson, OH 60089
614-555-0100

11/2/09
DATE

Cedera Lomos
PATIENT NAME

Dr. Katherine Yan
PROVIDER

LOMCE000
CHART #

OFFICE VISITS - SYMPTOMATIC	
99201	OF--New Patient Minimal
99202	OF--New Patient Low
99203	OF--New Patient Detailed
99204	OF--New Patient Moderate
99205	OF--New Patient High
99211	OF--Established Patient Minimal
99212	OF--Established Patient Low
99213	OF--Established Patient Detailed
99214	OF--Established Patient Moderate
99215	OF--Established Patient High

PREVENTIVE VISITS	
NEW	
99381	Under 1 Year
99382	1 - 4 Years
99383	5 - 11 Years
99384	12 - 17 Years
99385	18 - 39 Years
99386	40 - 64 Years
99387	65 Years & Up
ESTABLISHED	
99391	Under 1 Year
99392	1 - 4 Years
99393	5 - 11 Years
99394	12 - 17 Years
99395	18 - 39 Years
99396	40 - 64 Years
99397	65 Years & Up

PROCEDURES	
12011	Repair of superficial wounds, face
29125	Short arm splint
45378	Colonoscopy--diagnostic
45380	Colonoscopy--biopsy
71010	Chest x-ray, frontal
71020	Chest x-ray, frontal and lateral
73070	Elbow x-ray, AP and lateral

73090	Forearm x-ray, AP and lateral
73100	Wrist x-ray, AP and lateral
73600	Ankle x-ray, AP and lateral
93000	Electrocardiogram--EEG
93015	Treadmill stress test

LABORATORY	
80061	Lipid panel
82270	Hemoccult--stool screening
82465	Cholesterol test
82947	Glucose--quantitative
82951	Glucose tolerance test
83718	HDL cholesterol test
85007	Manual WBC
85025	CBC w/diff.
85651	Erythrocyte sed rate--ESR
86585	Tine test
87040	Strep culture
87430	Strep screen
87086	Urine colony count
87088	Urine culture

INJECTIONS	
90471	Immunization administration
90657	Influenza injection, under 35 months
90658	Influenza injection, older than 3 years
90703	Tetanus immunization
90707	MMR immunization

REFERRING PHYSICIAN

NPI

NOTES

AUTHORIZATION #

DIAGNOSIS
Chronic sinusitis

PAYMENT AMOUNT

Family Care Center
285 Stephenson Boulevard
Stephenson, OH 60089
614-555-0100

11/2/09
DATE

Stanley Feldman
PATIENT NAME

Dr. Katherine Yan
PROVIDER

FELST000
CHART #

OFFICE VISITS - SYMPTOMATIC	
99201	OF--New Patient Minimal
99202	OF--New Patient Low
99203	OF--New Patient Detailed
99204	OF--New Patient Moderate
99205	OF--New Patient High
99211	OF--Established Patient Minimal
99212	OF--Established Patient Low
99213	OF--Established Patient Detailed
99214	OF--Established Patient Moderate
99215	OF--Established Patient High
PREVENTIVE VISITS	
NEW	
99381	Under 1 Year
99382	1 - 4 Years
99383	5 - 11 Years
99384	12 - 17 Years
99385	18 - 39 Years
99386	40 - 64 Years
99387	65 Years & Up
ESTABLISHED	
99391	Under 1 Year
99392	1 - 4 Years
99393	5 - 11 Years
99394	12 - 17 Years
99395	18 - 39 Years
99396	40 - 64 Years
99397	65 Years & Up
PROCEDURES	
12011	Repair of superficial wounds, face
29125	Short arm splint
45378	Colonoscopy--diagnostic
45380	Colonoscopy--biopsy
71010	Chest x-ray, frontal
71020	Chest x-ray, frontal and lateral
73070	Elbow x-ray, AP and lateral

73090	Forearm x-ray, AP and lateral
73100	Wrist x-ray, AP and lateral
73600	Ankle x-ray, AP and lateral
93000	Electrocardiogram--EEG
93015	Treadmill stress test
LABORATORY	
80061	Lipid panel
82270	Hemoccult--stool screening
82465	Cholesterol test
82947	Glucose--quantitative
82951	Glucose tolerance test
83718	HDL cholesterol test
85007	Manual WBC
85025	CBC w/diff.
85651	Erythrocyte sed rate--ESR
86585	Tine test
87040	Strep culture
87430	Strep screen
87086	Urine colony count
87088	Urine culture
INJECTIONS	
90471	Immunization administration
90657	Influenza injection, under 35 months
90658	Influenza injection, older than 3 years
90703	Tetanus immunization
90707	MMR immunization

REFERRING PHYSICIAN

NPI

NOTES

AUTHORIZATION #

DIAGNOSIS

Hypercholesterolemia

PAYMENT AMOUNT

11/2/09
DATE

Ethan Sampson
PATIENT NAME

Family Care Center
285 Stephenson Boulevard
Stephenson, OH 60089
614-555-0100

Dr. Katherine Yan
PROVIDER

SAMET000
CHART #

OFFICE VISITS - SYMPTOMATIC	
99201	OF--New Patient Minimal
99202	OF--New Patient Low
99203	OF--New Patient Detailed
99204	OF--New Patient Moderate
99205	OF--New Patient High
99211	OF--Established Patient Minimal
99212	OF--Established Patient Low
99213	OF--Established Patient Detailed
99214	OF--Established Patient Moderate
99215	OF--Established Patient High
PREVENTIVE VISITS	
NEW	
99381	Under 1 Year
99382	1 - 4 Years
99383	5 - 11 Years
99384	12 - 17 Years
99385	18 - 39 Years
99386	40 - 64 Years
99387	65 Years & Up
ESTABLISHED	
99391	Under 1 Year
99392	1 - 4 Years
99393	5 - 11 Years
99394	12 - 17 Years
99395	18 - 39 Years
99396	40 - 64 Years
99397	65 Years & Up
PROCEDURES	
12011	Repair of superficial wounds, face
29125	Short arm splint
45378	Colonoscopy--diagnostic
45380	Colonoscopy--biopsy
71010	Chest x-ray, frontal
71020	Chest x-ray, frontal and lateral
73070	Elbow x-ray, AP and lateral

73090	Forearm x-ray, AP and lateral
73100	Wrist x-ray, AP and lateral
73600	Ankle x-ray, AP and lateral
93000	Electrocardiogram--EEG
93015	Treadmill stress test
LABORATORY	
80061	Lipid panel
82270	Hemoccult--stool screening
82465	Cholesterol test
82947	Glucose--quantitative
82951	Glucose tolerance test
83718	HDL cholesterol test
85007	Manual WBC
85025	CBC w/diff.
85651	Erythrocyte sed rate--ESR
86585	Tine test
87040	Strep culture
87430	Strep screen
87086	Urine colony count
87088	Urine culture
INJECTIONS	
90471	Immunization administration
90657	Influenza injection, under 35 months
90658	Influenza injection, older than 3 years
90703	Tetanus immunization
90707	MMR immunization

REFERRING PHYSICIAN

NPI

NOTES

AUTHORIZATION #

DIAGNOSIS
Sprain or strain

PAYMENT AMOUNT
$15 copayment, check #129

PATIENT INFORMATION FORM

THIS SECTION REFERS TO PATIENT ONLY			

Name: Jo Black	Sex: F	Marital Status: ☒S ☐M ☐D ☐W	Birth Date: 1/11/58

Address: 3 Parkway Road	SS#: 321-22-8787

City: Stephenson	State: OH	Zip: 60089	Employer: Barden Elementary School (full-time)

Home Phone: 614-555-8989	Employer's Address:

Work Phone: 614-879-2000	City:	State:	Zip:

Spouse's Name:	Spouse's Employer:

Emergency Contact:	Relationship:	Phone #:

FILL IN IF PATIENT IS A MINOR			

Parent/Guardian's Name:	Sex:	Marital Status: ☐S ☐M ☐D ☐W	Birth Date:

Phone:	SS#:

Address:	Employer:

City:	State:	Zip:	Employer's Address:

Student Status:	City:	State:	Zip:

INSURANCE INFORMATION	

Primary Insurance Company: Blue Cross/Blue Shield	Secondary Insurance Company:

Subscriber's Name: (same)	Birth Date: 1/11/58	Subscriber's Name:	Birth Date:

Plan:	SS#: 321-22-8787	Plan:

Policy #: 321228787	Group #: BE134	Policy #:	Group #:

Deductible $200	Price Code: A

OTHER INFORMATION	

Reason for visit:	Allergy to Medication (list):

Name of referring physician:	If auto accident, list date and state in which it occurred:

Regardless of any insurance coverage I may or may not have, it is my responsibility to pay the entire bill. In the event that this office needs to obtain legal assistance in collection of any unpaid balance, I agree to pay costs and attorney fees, as allowable by law. I authorize the release of the above patient's medical records for billing purposes. I authorize payment of medical benefits to Dr. Katherine Yan, Dr. Jessica Rudner, or Dr. John Rudner.

Jo Black	11/2/2009
(Patient's Signature/Parent or Guardian's Signature)	(Date)

11/2/09
DATE

Family Care Center
285 Stephenson Boulevard
Stephenson, OH 60089
614-555-0100

Dr. Katherine Yan
PROVIDER

Jo Black
PATIENT NAME

BLAJO000
CHART #

OFFICE VISITS - SYMPTOMATIC	
99201	OF--New Patient Minimal
99202	OF--New Patient Low
99203	OF--New Patient Detailed
99204	OF--New Patient Moderate
99205	OF--New Patient High
99211	OF--Established Patient Minimal
99212	OF--Established Patient Low
99213	OF--Established Patient Detailed
99214	OF--Established Patient Moderate
99215	OF--Established Patient High

PREVENTIVE VISITS	
NEW	
99381	Under 1 Year
99382	1 - 4 Years
99383	5 - 11 Years
99384	12 - 17 Years
99385	18 - 39 Years
99386	40 - 64 Years
99387	65 Years & Up
ESTABLISHED	
99391	Under 1 Year
99392	1 - 4 Years
99393	5 - 11 Years
99394	12 - 17 Years
99395	18 - 39 Years
99396	40 - 64 Years
99397	65 Years & Up

PROCEDURES	
12011	Repair of superficial wounds, face
29125	Short arm splint
45378	Colonoscopy--diagnostic
45380	Colonoscopy--biopsy
71010	Chest x-ray, frontal
71020	Chest x-ray, frontal and lateral
73070	Elbow x-ray, AP and lateral

73090	Forearm x-ray, AP and lateral
73100	Wrist x-ray, AP and lateral
73600	Ankle x-ray, AP and lateral
93000	Electrocardiogram--EEG
93015	Treadmill stress test

LABORATORY	
80061	Lipid panel
82270	Hemoccult--stool screening
82465	Cholesterol test
82947	Glucose--quantitative
82951	Glucose tolerance test
83718	HDL cholesterol test
85007	Manual WBC
85025	CBC w/diff.
85651	Erythrocyte sed rate--ESR
86585	Tine test
87040	Strep culture
87430	Strep screen
87086	Urine colony count
87088	Urine culture

INJECTIONS	
90471	Immunization administration
90657	Influenza injection, under 35 months
90658	Influenza injection, older than 3 years
90703	Tetanus immunization
90707	MMR immunization

REFERRING PHYSICIAN

NPI

NOTES

AUTHORIZATION #

DIAGNOSIS
Arrhythmia

PAYMENT AMOUNT

Family Care Center
285 Stephenson Boulevard
Stephenson, OH 60089
614-555-0100

11/2/09
DATE

Sarina Bell
PATIENT NAME

Dr. Katherine Yan
PROVIDER

BELSA001
CHART #

OFFICE VISITS - SYMPTOMATIC	
99201	OF--New Patient Minimal
99202	OF--New Patient Low
99203	OF--New Patient Detailed
99204	OF--New Patient Moderate
99205	OF--New Patient High
99211	OF--Established Patient Minimal
99212	OF--Established Patient Low
99213	OF--Established Patient Detailed
99214	OF--Established Patient Moderate
99215	OF--Established Patient High
PREVENTIVE VISITS	
NEW	
99381	Under 1 Year
99382	1 - 4 Years
99383	5 - 11 Years
99384	12 - 17 Years
99385	18 - 39 Years
99386	40 - 64 Years
99387	65 Years & Up
ESTABLISHED	
99391	Under 1 Year
99392	1 - 4 Years
99393	5 - 11 Years
99394	12 - 17 Years
99395	18 - 39 Years
99396	40 - 64 Years
99397	65 Years & Up
PROCEDURES	
12011	Repair of superficial wounds, face
29125	Short arm splint
45378	Colonoscopy--diagnostic
45380	Colonoscopy--biopsy
71010	Chest x-ray, frontal
71020	Chest x-ray, frontal and lateral
73070	Elbow x-ray, AP and lateral

73090	Forearm x-ray, AP and lateral
73100	Wrist x-ray, AP and lateral
73600	Ankle x-ray, AP and lateral
93000	Electrocardiogram--EEG
93015	Treadmill stress test
LABORATORY	
80061	Lipid panel
82270	Hemoccult--stool screening
82465	Cholesterol test
82947	Glucose--quantitative
82951	Glucose tolerance test
83718	HDL cholesterol test
85007	Manual WBC
85025	CBC w/diff.
85651	Erythrocyte sed rate--ESR
86585	Tine test
87040	Strep culture
87430	Strep screen
87086	Urine colony count
87088	Urine culture
INJECTIONS	
90471	Immunization administration
90657	Influenza injection, under 35 months
90658	Influenza injection, older than 3 years
90703	Tetanus immunization
90707	MMR immunization

REFERRING PHYSICIAN   NPI

AUTHORIZATION #

NOTES

DIAGNOSIS
Laceration of eyelid
PAYMENT AMOUNT
$15 copayment, check #1421

TRICARE
249 Center Street
Columbus, OH 60220

PROVIDER REMITTANCE
THIS IS NOT A BILL
A PAYMENT SUMMARY AND AN EXPLANATION OF
CODES ARE AT THE END OF THIS STATEMENT

FAMILY CARE CENTER
285 STEPHENSON BLVD.
STEPHENSON, OH 60089

PAGE: 1 OF 1
DATE: 11/2/09
ID NUMBER: 7394578

PROVIDER: KATHERINE YAN, M.D.

PATIENT: TANAKA HIRO

PROC CODE	FROM DATE	THRU DATE	TREAT -MENT	STATUS CODE	AMOUNT CHRGD	AMOUNT ALLWD	COPAY/ DEDUCT	AMOUNT APPRVD	PATIENT BALANCE
99212	8/12/09	8/12/09	1	A	28.00	28.00	10.00	28.00	.00
73600	8/12/09	8/12/09	1	A	27.00	27.00	.00	27.00	.00
99212	8/18/09	8/18/09	1	A	28.00	28.00	10.00	28.00	.00
99212	9/4/09	9/4/09	1	A	28.00	28.00	10.00	28.00	.00
		TOTALS			111.00	111.00	30.00	111.00	.00

PATIENT: PETERSON ANN

PROC CODE	FROM DATE	THRU DATE	TREAT -MENT	STATUS CODE	AMOUNT CHRGD	AMOUNT ALLWD	COPAY/ DEDUCT	AMOUNT APPRVD	PATIENT BALANCE
99201	7/20/09	7/20/09	1	A	32.00	32.00	10.00	32.00	.00
		TOTALS			32.00	32.00	10.00	32.00	.00

PAYMENT SUMMARY

TOTAL AMOUNT PAID	143.00
PRIOR CREDIT BALANCE	.00
CURRENT CREDIT DEFERRED	.00
PRIOR CREDIT APPLIED	.00
NEW CREDIT BALANCE	.00
NET DISBURSED	143.00

TOTAL ALL CLAIMS

AMOUNT CHARGES	143.00
AMOUNT ALLOWED	143.00
DEDUCTIBLE	.00
COPAY	40.00
OTHER REDUCTION	.00
AMOUNT APPROVED	143.00

EFT INFORMATION

NUMBER	7394578
DATE	11/2/09
AMOUNT	143.00

STATUS CODES:
A - APPROVED   AJ - ADJUSTMENT   IP - IN PROCESS   R - REJECTED   V - VOID

11/4/09
DATE

Family Care Center
285 Stephenson Boulevard
Stephenson, OH 60089
614-555-0100

Dr. Katherine Yan
PROVIDER

John Gardiner
PATIENT NAME

GARJO000
CHART #

OFFICE VISITS - SYMPTOMATIC	
99201	OF--New Patient Minimal
99202	OF--New Patient Low
99203	OF--New Patient Detailed
99204	OF--New Patient Moderate
99205	OF--New Patient High
99211	OF--Established Patient Minimal
99212	OF--Established Patient Low
99213	OF--Established Patient Detailed
99214	OF--Established Patient Moderate
99215	OF--Established Patient High

PREVENTIVE VISITS	
NEW	
99381	Under 1 Year
99382	1 - 4 Years
99383	5 - 11 Years
99384	12 - 17 Years
99385	18 - 39 Years
99386	40 - 64 Years
99387	65 Years & Up
ESTABLISHED	
99391	Under 1 Year
99392	1 - 4 Years
99393	5 - 11 Years
99394	12 - 17 Years
99395	18 - 39 Years
99396	40 - 64 Years
99397	65 Years & Up

PROCEDURES	
12011	Repair of superficial wounds, face
29125	Short arm splint
45378	Colonoscopy--diagnostic
45380	Colonoscopy--biopsy
71010	Chest x-ray, frontal
71020	Chest x-ray, frontal and lateral
73070	Elbow x-ray, AP and lateral

73090	Forearm x-ray, AP and lateral
73100	Wrist x-ray, AP and lateral
73600	Ankle x-ray, AP and lateral
93000	Electrocardiogram--EEG
93015	Treadmill stress test

LABORATORY	
80061	Lipid panel
82270	Hemoccult--stool screening
82465	Cholesterol test
82947	Glucose--quantitative
82951	Glucose tolerance test
83718	HDL cholesterol test
85007	Manual WBC
85025	CBC w/diff.
85651	Erythrocyte sed rate--ESR
86585	Tine test
87040	Strep culture
87430	Strep screen
87086	Urine colony count
87088	Urine culture

INJECTIONS	
90471	Immunization administration
90657	Influenza injection, under 35 months
90658	Influenza injection, older than 3 years
90703	Tetanus immunization
90707	MMR immunization

REFERRING PHYSICIAN

NPI

NOTES

AUTHORIZATION #

DIAGNOSIS
Influenza

PAYMENT AMOUNT
$15 copayment, check #2327

Family Care Center
285 Stephenson Boulevard
Stephenson, OH 60089
614-555-0100

Things to Do Today

Date 11/4/2009

Patient Paul Ramos

Paul Ramos has a new home telephone number:

614-332-4398

PATIENT INFORMATION FORM

THIS SECTION REFERS TO PATIENT ONLY

Name: Sam Wu	Sex: M	Marital Status: ☐S ☐M ☒D ☐W	Birth Date: 8/8/52

Address: 4701 Plymouth Avenue	SS#: 381-77-9138

City: Stephenson	State: OH	Zip: 60089	Employer: Stephenson Construction (full-time)

Home Phone: 614-931-3319	Employer's Address:

Work Phone: 614-555-3211	City:	State:	Zip:

Spouse's Name:	Spouse's Employer:

Emergency Contact:	Relationship:	Phone #:

FILL IN IF PATIENT IS A MINOR

Parent/Guardian's Name:	Sex:	Marital Status: ☐S ☐M ☐D ☐W	Birth Date:

Phone:	SS#:

Address:	Employer:

City:	State:	Zip:	Employer's Address:

Student Status:	City:	State:	Zip:

INSURANCE INFORMATION

Primary Insurance Company: U.S. Life	Secondary Insurance Company:

Subscriber's Name: (same)	Birth Date: 8/8/52	Subscriber's Name:	Birth Date:

Plan:	SS#: 381-77-9138	Plan:

Policy #: 381779138	Group #: 931	Policy #:	Group #:

Copayment: $15	Price Code: B

OTHER INFORMATION

Reason for visit: Arm hurts when moved	Allergy to Medication (list):

Name of referring physician:	If auto accident, list date and state in which it occurred: 11/1/2009, OH

Regardless of any insurance coverage I may or may not have, it is my responsibility to pay the entire bill. In the event that this office needs to obtain legal assistance in collection of any unpaid balance, I agree to pay costs and attorney fees, as allowable by law. I authorize the release of the above patient's medical records for billing purposes. I authorize payment of medical benefits to Dr. Katherine Yan, Dr. Jessica Rudner, or Dr. John Rudner.

Sam Wu   11/4/2009

(Patient's Signature/Parent or Guardian's Signature)   (Date)

11/4/09
DATE

Family Care Center
285 Stephenson Boulevard
Stephenson, OH 60089
614-555-0100

Dr. Katherine Yan
PROVIDER

Sam Wu
PATIENT NAME

WUSA0000
CHART #

OFFICE VISITS - SYMPTOMATIC	
99201	OF--New Patient Minimal
99202	OF--New Patient Low
99203	OF--New Patient Detailed
99204	OF--New Patient Moderate
99205	OF--New Patient High
99211	OF--Established Patient Minimal
99212	OF--Established Patient Low
99213	OF--Established Patient Detailed
99214	OF--Established Patient Moderate
99215	OF--Established Patient High
PREVENTIVE VISITS	
NEW	
99381	Under 1 Year
99382	1 - 4 Years
99383	5 - 11 Years
99384	12 - 17 Years
99385	18 - 39 Years
99386	40 - 64 Years
99387	65 Years & Up
ESTABLISHED	
99391	Under 1 Year
99392	1 - 4 Years
99393	5 - 11 Years
99394	12 - 17 Years
99395	18 - 39 Years
99396	40 - 64 Years
99397	65 Years & Up
PROCEDURES	
12011	Repair of superficial wounds, face
29125	Short arm splint
45378	Colonoscopy--diagnostic
45380	Colonoscopy--biopsy
71010	Chest x-ray, frontal
71020	Chest x-ray, frontal and lateral
73070	Elbow x-ray, AP and lateral

73090	Forearm x-ray, AP and lateral
73100	Wrist x-ray, AP and lateral
73600	Ankle x-ray, AP and lateral
93000	Electrocardiogram--EEG
93015	Treadmill stress test
LABORATORY	
80061	Lipid panel
82270	Hemoccult--stool screening
82465	Cholesterol test
82947	Glucose--quantitative
82951	Glucose tolerance test
83718	HDL cholesterol test
85007	Manual WBC
85025	CBC w/diff.
85651	Erythrocyte sed rate--ESR
86585	Tine test
87040	Strep culture
87430	Strep screen
87086	Urine colony count
87088	Urine culture
INJECTIONS	
90471	Immunization administration
90657	Influenza injection, under 35 months
90658	Influenza injection, older than 3 years
90703	Tetanus immunization
90707	MMR immunization

REFERRING PHYSICIAN

NPI

NOTES

AUTHORIZATION #

DIAGNOSIS
Sprain or strain

PAYMENT AMOUNT
$15 copayment, check #561

Family Care Center
285 Stephenson Boulevard
Stephenson, OH 60089
614-555-0100

11/4/09
DATE

Paul Ramos
PATIENT NAME

Dr. Katherine Yan
PROVIDER

RAMPA000
CHART #

OFFICE VISITS - SYMPTOMATIC	
99201	OF--New Patient Minimal
99202	OF--New Patient Low
99203	OF--New Patient Detailed
99204	OF--New Patient Moderate
99205	OF--New Patient High
99211	OF--Established Patient Minimal
99212	OF--Established Patient Low
99213	OF--Established Patient Detailed
99214	OF--Established Patient Moderate
99215	OF--Established Patient High

PREVENTIVE VISITS	
NEW	
99381	Under 1 Year
99382	1 - 4 Years
99383	5 - 11 Years
99384	12 - 17 Years
99385	18 - 39 Years
99386	40 - 64 Years
99387	65 Years & Up
ESTABLISHED	
99391	Under 1 Year
99392	1 - 4 Years
99393	5 - 11 Years
99394	12 - 17 Years
99395	18 - 39 Years
99396	40 - 64 Years
99397	65 Years & Up

PROCEDURES	
12011	Repair of superficial wounds, face
29125	Short arm splint
45378	Colonoscopy--diagnostic
45380	Colonoscopy--biopsy
71010	Chest x-ray, frontal
71020	Chest x-ray, frontal and lateral
73070	Elbow x-ray, AP and lateral

73090	Forearm x-ray, AP and lateral
73100	Wrist x-ray, AP and lateral
73600	Ankle x-ray, AP and lateral
93000	Electrocardiogram--EEG
93015	Treadmill stress test

LABORATORY	
80061	Lipid panel
82270	Hemoccult--stool screening
82465	Cholesterol test
82947	Glucose--quantitative
82951	Glucose tolerance test
83718	HDL cholesterol test
85007	Manual WBC
85025	CBC w/diff.
85651	Erythrocyte sed rate--ESR
86585	Tine test
87040	Strep culture
87430	Strep screen
87086	Urine colony count
87088	Urine culture

INJECTIONS	
90471	Immunization administration
90657	Influenza injection, under 35 months
90658	Influenza injection, older than 3 years
90703	Tetanus immunization
90707	MMR immunization

REFERRING PHYSICIAN

NPI

NOTES

AUTHORIZATION #

DIAGNOSIS
Urinary tract infection

PAYMENT AMOUNT
$15 copayment, check #2011

11/4/09
DATE

Family Care Center
285 Stephenson Boulevard
Stephenson, OH 60089
614-555-0100

Dr. Katherine Yan
PROVIDER

Ellen Barmenstein
PATIENT NAME

BAREL000
CHART #

OFFICE VISITS - SYMPTOMATIC	
99201	OF--New Patient Minimal
99202	OF--New Patient Low
99203	OF--New Patient Detailed
99204	OF--New Patient Moderate
99205	OF--New Patient High
99211	OF--Established Patient Minimal
99212	OF--Established Patient Low
99213	OF--Established Patient Detailed
99214	OF--Established Patient Moderate
99215	OF--Established Patient High
PREVENTIVE VISITS	
NEW	
99381	Under 1 Year
99382	1 - 4 Years
99383	5 - 11 Years
99384	12 - 17 Years
99385	18 - 39 Years
99386	40 - 64 Years
99387	65 Years & Up
ESTABLISHED	
99391	Under 1 Year
99392	1 - 4 Years
99393	5 - 11 Years
99394	12 - 17 Years
99395	18 - 39 Years
99396	40 - 64 Years
99397	65 Years & Up
PROCEDURES	
12011	Repair of superficial wounds, face
29125	Short arm splint
45378	Colonoscopy--diagnostic
45380	Colonoscopy--biopsy
71010	Chest x-ray, frontal
71020	Chest x-ray, frontal and lateral
73070	Elbow x-ray, AP and lateral

73090	Forearm x-ray, AP and lateral
73100	Wrist x-ray, AP and lateral
73600	Ankle x-ray, AP and lateral
93000	Electrocardiogram--EEG
93015	Treadmill stress test
LABORATORY	
80061	Lipid panel
82270	Hemoccult--stool screening
82465	Cholesterol test
82947	Glucose--quantitative
82951	Glucose tolerance test
83718	HDL cholesterol test
85007	Manual WBC
85025	CBC w/diff.
85651	Erythrocyte sed rate--ESR
86585	Tine test
87040	Strep culture
87430	Strep screen
87086	Urine colony count
87088	Urine culture
INJECTIONS	
90471	Immunization administration
90657	Influenza injection, under 35 months
90658	Influenza injection, older than 3 years
90703	Tetanus immunization
90707	MMR immunization

REFERRING PHYSICIAN   NPI

NOTES

AUTHORIZATION #

DIAGNOSIS
Hypercholesterolemia
PAYMENT AMOUNT

11/4/09
DATE

Family Care Center
285 Stephenson Boulevard
Stephenson, OH 60089
614-555-0100

Dr. Katherine Yan
PROVIDER

Jones, Elizabeth
PATIENT NAME

JONEL000
CHART #

OFFICE VISITS - SYMPTOMATIC	
99201	OF--New Patient Minimal
99202	OF--New Patient Low
99203	OF--New Patient Detailed
99204	OF--New Patient Moderate
99205	OF--New Patient High
99211	OF--Established Patient Minimal
99212	OF--Established Patient Low
99213	OF--Established Patient Detailed
99214	OF--Established Patient Moderate
99215	OF--Established Patient High

PREVENTIVE VISITS	
NEW	
99381	Under 1 Year
99382	1 - 4 Years
99383	5 - 11 Years
99384	12 - 17 Years
99385	18 - 39 Years
99386	40 - 64 Years
99387	65 Years & Up

ESTABLISHED	
99391	Under 1 Year
99392	1 - 4 Years
99393	5 - 11 Years
99394	12 - 17 Years
99395	18 - 39 Years
99396	40 - 64 Years
99397	65 Years & Up

PROCEDURES	
12011	Repair of superficial wounds, face
29125	Short arm splint
45378	Colonoscopy--diagnostic
45380	Colonoscopy--biopsy
71010	Chest x-ray, frontal
71020	Chest x-ray, frontal and lateral
73070	Elbow x-ray, AP and lateral

73090	Forearm x-ray, AP and lateral
73100	Wrist x-ray, AP and lateral
73600	Ankle x-ray, AP and lateral
93000	Electrocardiogram--EEG
93015	Treadmill stress test

LABORATORY	
80061	Lipid panel
82270	Hemoccult--stool screening
82465	Cholesterol test
82947	Glucose--quantitative
82951	Glucose tolerance test
83718	HDL cholesterol test
85007	Manual WBC
85025	CBC w/diff.
85651	Erythrocyte sed rate--ESR
86585	Tine test
87040	Strep culture
87430	Strep screen
87086	Urine colony count
87088	Urine culture

INJECTIONS◦	
90471	Immunization administration
90657	Influenza injection, under 35 months
90658	Influenza injection, older than 3 years
90703	Tetanus immunization
90707	MMR immunization

REFERRING PHYSICIAN	NPI	NOTES
AUTHORIZATION #		

DIAGNOSIS
Laceration

PAYMENT AMOUNT
$15 copayment, check #4226

Family Care Center
285 Stephenson Boulevard
Stephenson, OH 60089
614-555-0100

11/4/09
DATE

Smith, James L.
PATIENT NAME

Dr. Katherine Yan
PROVIDER

SMIJA000
CHART #

OFFICE VISITS - SYMPTOMATIC	
99201	OF--New Patient Minimal
99202	OF--New Patient Low
99203	OF--New Patient Detailed
99204	OF--New Patient Moderate
99205	OF--New Patient High
99211	OF--Established Patient Minimal
99212	OF--Established Patient Low
99213	OF--Established Patient Detailed
99214	OF--Established Patient Moderate
99215	OF--Established Patient High
PREVENTIVE VISITS	
NEW	
99381	Under 1 Year
99382	1 - 4 Years
99383	5 - 11 Years
99384	12 - 17 Years
99385	18 - 39 Years
99386	40 - 64 Years
99387	65 Years & Up
ESTABLISHED	
99391	Under 1 Year
99392	1 - 4 Years
99393	5 - 11 Years
99394	12 - 17 Years
99395	18 - 39 Years
99396	40 - 64 Years
99397	65 Years & Up
PROCEDURES	
12011	Repair of superficial wounds, face
29125	Short arm splint
45378	Colonoscopy--diagnostic
45380	Colonoscopy--biopsy
71010	Chest x-ray, frontal
71020	Chest x-ray, frontal and lateral
73070	Elbow x-ray, AP and lateral

73090	Forearm x-ray, AP and lateral
73100	Wrist x-ray, AP and lateral
73600	Ankle x-ray, AP and lateral
93000	Electrocardiogram--EEG
93015	Treadmill stress test
LABORATORY	
80061	Lipid panel
82270	Hemoccult--stool screening
82465	Cholesterol test
82947	Glucose--quantitative
82951	Glucose tolerance test
83718	HDL cholesterol test
85007	Manual WBC
85025	CBC w/diff.
85651	Erythrocyte sed rate--ESR
86585	Tine test
87040	Strep culture
87430	Strep screen
87086	Urine colony count
87088	Urine culture
INJECTIONS	
90471	Immunization administration
90657	Influenza injection, under 35 months
90658	Influenza injection, older than 3 years
90703	Tetanus immunization
90707	MMR immunization

REFERRING PHYSICIAN

NPI

NOTES

AUTHORIZATION #

DIAGNOSIS
Pain - chest

PAYMENT AMOUNT

PATIENT INFORMATION FORM

THIS SECTION REFERS TO PATIENT ONLY

Name: Joe Abate		Sex: M	Marital Status: ☐S ☒M ☐D ☐W	Birth Date: 10/1/67

Address: 86 Western Drive

SS#: 403-53-3491

City: Stephenson	State: OH	Zip: 60089	Employer: Stephenson Wire Works (full-time)

Home Phone: 614-931-3317

Employer's Address:

Work Phone: 614-525-0215

City: State: Zip:

Spouse's Name:

Spouse's Employer:

Emergency Contact:

Relationship: Phone #:

FILL IN IF PATIENT IS A MINOR

Parent/Guardian's Name:

Sex: Marital Status: ☐S ☐M ☐D ☐W   Birth Date:

Phone:

SS#:

Address:

Employer:

City: State: Zip:

Employer's Address:

Student Status:

City: State: Zip:

INSURANCE INFORMATION

Primary Insurance Company: Physician's Choice

Secondary Insurance Company:

Subscriber's Name: (same)   Birth Date: 10/1/67

Subscriber's Name: Birth Date:

Plan: SS#: 403-53-3491

Plan:

Policy #: 321728   Group #: E4362

Policy #:   Group #:

Copayment: $15   Price Code: B

OTHER INFORMATION

Reason for visit: Preventive exam

Allergy to Medication (list):

Name of referring physician:

If auto accident, list date and state in which it occurred:

Regardless of any insurance coverage I may or may not have, it is my responsibility to pay the entire bill. In the event that this office needs to obtain legal assistance in collection of any unpaid balance, I agree to pay costs and attorney fees, as allowable by law. I authorize the release of the above patient's medical records for billing purposes. I authorize payment of medical benefits to Dr. Katherine Yan, Dr. Jessica Rudner, or Dr. John Rudner.

Joe Abate   11/4/2009

(Patient's Signature/Parent or Guardian's Signature)   (Date)

Family Care Center
285 Stephenson Boulevard
Stephenson, OH 60089
614-555-0100

11/4/09
DATE

Abate, Joe
PATIENT NAME

Dr. Katherine Yan
PROVIDER

ABAJO000
CHART #

OFFICE VISITS - SYMPTOMATIC	
99201	OF--New Patient Minimal
99202	OF--New Patient Low
99203	OF--New Patient Detailed
99204	OF--New Patient Moderate
99205	OF--New Patient High
99211	OF--Established Patient Minimal
99212	OF--Established Patient Low
99213	OF--Established Patient Detailed
99214	OF--Established Patient Moderate
99215	OF--Established Patient High
PREVENTIVE VISITS	
NEW	
99381	Under 1 Year
99382	1 - 4 Years
99383	5 - 11 Years
99384	12 - 17 Years
99385	18 - 39 Years
99386	40 - 64 Years
99387	65 Years & Up
ESTABLISHED	
99391	Under 1 Year
99392	1 - 4 Years
99393	5 - 11 Years
99394	12 - 17 Years
99395	18 - 39 Years
99396	40 - 64 Years
99397	65 Years & Up
PROCEDURES	
12011	Repair of superficial wounds, face
29125	Short arm splint
45378	Colonoscopy--diagnostic
45380	Colonoscopy--biopsy
71010	Chest x-ray, frontal
71020	Chest x-ray, frontal and lateral
73070	Elbow x-ray, AP and lateral

73090	Forearm x-ray, AP and lateral
73100	Wrist x-ray, AP and lateral
73600	Ankle x-ray, AP and lateral
93000	Electrocardiogram--EEG
93015	Treadmill stress test
LABORATORY	
80061	Lipid panel
82270	Hemoccult--stool screening
82465	Cholesterol test
82947	Glucose--quantitative
82951	Glucose tolerance test
83718	HDL cholesterol test
85007	Manual WBC
85025	CBC w/diff.
85651	Erythrocyte sed rate--ESR
86585	Tine test
87040	Strep culture
87430	Strep screen
87086	Urine colony count
87088	Urine culture
INJECTIONS	
90471	Immunization administration
90657	Influenza injection, under 35 months
90658	Influenza injection, older than 3 years
90703	Tetanus immunization
90707	MMR immunization

REFERRING PHYSICIAN

NPI

NOTES

AUTHORIZATION #

DIAGNOSIS
Routine physical exam

PAYMENT AMOUNT
$15 copayment, check #124

11/4/09
DATE

Smith, Sarabeth
PATIENT NAME

Family Care Center
285 Stephenson Boulevard
Stephenson, OH 60089
614-555-0100

Dr. Katherine Yan
PROVIDER

SMISA000
CHART #

OFFICE VISITS - SYMPTOMATIC	
99201	OF--New Patient Minimal
99202	OF--New Patient Low
99203	OF--New Patient Detailed
99204	OF--New Patient Moderate
99205	OF--New Patient High
99211	OF--Established Patient Minimal
99212	OF--Established Patient Low
99213	OF--Established Patient Detailed
99214	OF--Established Patient Moderate
99215	OF--Established Patient High

PREVENTIVE VISITS	
NEW	
99381	Under 1 Year
99382	1 - 4 Years
99383	5 - 11 Years
99384	12 - 17 Years
99385	18 - 39 Years
99386	40 - 64 Years
99387	65 Years & Up
ESTABLISHED	
99391	Under 1 Year
99392	1 - 4 Years
99393	5 - 11 Years
99394	12 - 17 Years
99395	18 - 39 Years
99396	40 - 64 Years
99397	65 Years & Up

PROCEDURES	
12011	Repair of superficial wounds, face
29125	Short arm splint
45378	Colonoscopy--diagnostic
45380	Colonoscopy--biopsy
71010	Chest x-ray, frontal
71020	Chest x-ray, frontal and lateral
73070	Elbow x-ray, AP and lateral

73090	Forearm x-ray, AP and lateral
73100	Wrist x-ray, AP and lateral
73600	Ankle x-ray, AP and lateral
93000	Electrocardiogram--EEG
93015	Treadmill stress test

LABORATORY	
80061	Lipid panel
82270	Hemoccult--stool screening
82465	Cholesterol test
82947	Glucose--quantitative
82951	Glucose tolerance test
83718	HDL cholesterol test
85007	Manual WBC
85025	CBC w/diff.
85651	Erythrocyte sed rate--ESR
86585	Tine test
87040	Strep culture
87430	Strep screen
87086	Urine colony count
87088	Urine culture

INJECTIONS	
90471	Immunization administration
90657	Influenza injection, under 35 months
90658	Influenza injection, older than 3 years
90703	Tetanus immunization
90707	MMR immunization

REFERRING PHYSICIAN

NPI

NOTES

AUTHORIZATION #

DIAGNOSIS
Routine physical exam
PAYMENT AMOUNT

MARION JOHNSON
3511 WEST STREET
STEPHENSON OH 60089

No. 1234

Date Oct. 30, 2009

PAYABLE TO   Family Care Center

$61.20

Sixty-one and 20/100 ———————————————————————————— dollars

Stephenson Bank
Stephenson, OH 60089

Marion Johnson

021203347   0379 399 34   1234

11/5/09
DATE

Family Care Center
285 Stephenson Boulevard
Stephenson, OH 60089
614-555-0100

Dr. Katherine Yan
PROVIDER

Ramos, Maritza
PATIENT NAME

RAMMA000
CHART #

OFFICE VISITS - SYMPTOMATIC	
99201	OF--New Patient Minimal
99202	OF--New Patient Low
99203	OF--New Patient Detailed
99204	OF--New Patient Moderate
99205	OF--New Patient High
99211	OF--Established Patient Minimal
99212	OF--Established Patient Low
99213	OF--Established Patient Detailed
99214	OF--Established Patient Moderate
99215	OF--Established Patient High
PREVENTIVE VISITS	
NEW	
99381	Under 1 Year
99382	1 - 4 Years
99383	5 - 11 Years
99384	12 - 17 Years
99385	18 - 39 Years
99386	40 - 64 Years
99387	65 Years & Up
ESTABLISHED	
99391	Under 1 Year
99392	1 - 4 Years
99393	5 - 11 Years
99394	12 - 17 Years
99395	18 - 39 Years
99396	40 - 64 Years
99397	65 Years & Up
PROCEDURES	
12011	Repair of superficial wounds, face
29125	Short arm splint
45378	Colonoscopy--diagnostic
45380	Colonoscopy--biopsy
71010	Chest x-ray, frontal
71020	Chest x-ray, frontal and lateral
73070	Elbow x-ray, AP and lateral

73090	Forearm x-ray, AP and lateral
73100	Wrist x-ray, AP and lateral
73600	Ankle x-ray, AP and lateral
93000	Electrocardiogram--EEG
93015	Treadmill stress test
LABORATORY	
80061	Lipid panel
82270	Hemoccult--stool screening
82465	Cholesterol test
82947	Glucose--quantitative
82951	Glucose tolerance test
83718	HDL cholesterol test
85007	Manual WBC
85025	CBC w/diff.
85651	Erythrocyte sed rate--ESR
86585	Tine test
87040	Strep culture
87430	Strep screen
87086	Urine colony count
87088	Urine culture
INJECTIONS	
90471	Immunization administration
90657	Influenza injection, under 35 months
90658	Influenza injection, older than 3 years
90703	Tetanus immunization
90707	MMR immunization

REFERRING PHYSICIAN

NPI

NOTES

AUTHORIZATION #

DIAGNOSIS
Influenza

PAYMENT AMOUNT
$15 copayment, check #1047

11/5/09
DATE

Family Care Center
285 Stephenson Boulevard
Stephenson, OH 60089
614-555-0100

Dr. Katherine Yan
PROVIDER

Bell, Sarina
PATIENT NAME

BELSA000
CHART #

OFFICE VISITS - SYMPTOMATIC	
99201	OF--New Patient Minimal
99202	OF--New Patient Low
99203	OF--New Patient Detailed
99204	OF--New Patient Moderate
99205	OF--New Patient High
99211	OF--Established Patient Minimal
99212	OF--Established Patient Low
99213	OF--Established Patient Detailed
99214	OF--Established Patient Moderate
99215	OF--Established Patient High
PREVENTIVE VISITS	
NEW	
99381	Under 1 Year
99382	1 - 4 Years
99383	5 - 11 Years
99384	12 - 17 Years
99385	18 - 39 Years
99386	40 - 64 Years
99387	65 Years & Up
ESTABLISHED	
99391	Under 1 Year
99392	1 - 4 Years
99393	5 - 11 Years
99394	12 - 17 Years
99395	18 - 39 Years
99396	40 - 64 Years
99397	65 Years & Up
PROCEDURES	
12011	Repair of superficial wounds, face
29125	Short arm splint
45378	Colonoscopy--diagnostic
45380	Colonoscopy--biopsy
71010	Chest x-ray, frontal
71020	Chest x-ray, frontal and lateral
73070	Elbow x-ray, AP and lateral

73090	Forearm x-ray, AP and lateral
73100	Wrist x-ray, AP and lateral
73600	Ankle x-ray, AP and lateral
93000	Electrocardiogram--EEG
93015	Treadmill stress test
LABORATORY	
80061	Lipid panel
82270	Hemoccult--stool screening
82465	Cholesterol test
82947	Glucose--quantitative
82951	Glucose tolerance test
83718	HDL cholesterol test
85007	Manual WBC
85025	CBC w/diff.
85651	Erythrocyte sed rate--ESR
86585	Tine test
87040	Strep culture
87430	Strep screen
87086	Urine colony count
87088	Urine culture
INJECTIONS	
90471	Immunization administration
90657	Influenza injection, under 35 months
90658	Influenza injection, older than 3 years
90703	Tetanus immunization
90707	MMR immunization

REFERRING PHYSICIAN

NPI

NOTES

AUTHORIZATION #

DIAGNOSIS
Acute sinusitis

PAYMENT AMOUNT
$15 copayment, check #3126

Family Care Center
285 Stephenson Boulevard
Stephenson, OH 60089
614-555-0100

11/5/09
DATE

Wong, Jo
PATIENT NAME

Dr. Katherine Yan
PROVIDER

WONJO000
CHART #

OFFICE VISITS - SYMPTOMATIC	
99201	OF--New Patient Minimal
99202	OF--New Patient Low
99203	OF--New Patient Detailed
99204	OF--New Patient Moderate
99205	OF--New Patient High
99211	OF--Established Patient Minimal
99212	OF--Established Patient Low
99213	OF--Established Patient Detailed
99214	OF--Established Patient Moderate
99215	OF--Established Patient High

PREVENTIVE VISITS	
NEW	
99381	Under 1 Year
99382	1 - 4 Years
99383	5 - 11 Years
99384	12 - 17 Years
99385	18 - 39 Years
99386	40 - 64 Years
99387	65 Years & Up
ESTABLISHED	
99391	Under 1 Year
99392	1 - 4 Years
99393	5 - 11 Years
99394	12 - 17 Years
99395	18 - 39 Years
99396	40 - 64 Years
99397	65 Years & Up

PROCEDURES	
12011	Repair of superficial wounds, face
29125	Short arm splint
45378	Colonoscopy--diagnostic
45380	Colonoscopy--biopsy
71010	Chest x-ray, frontal
71020	Chest x-ray, frontal and lateral
73070	Elbow x-ray, AP and lateral

73090	Forearm x-ray, AP and lateral
73100	Wrist x-ray, AP and lateral
73600	Ankle x-ray, AP and lateral
93000	Electrocardiogram--EEG
93015	Treadmill stress test

LABORATORY	
80061	Lipid panel
82270	Hemoccult--stool screening
82465	Cholesterol test
82947	Glucose--quantitative
82951	Glucose tolerance test
83718	HDL cholesterol test
85007	Manual WBC
85025	CBC w/diff.
85651	Erythrocyte sed rate--ESR
86585	Tine test
87040	Strep culture
87430	Strep screen
87086	Urine colony count
87088	Urine culture

INJECTIONS	
90471	Immunization administration
90657	Influenza injection, under 35 months
90658	Influenza injection, older than 3 years
90703	Tetanus immunization
90707	MMR immunization

REFERRING PHYSICIAN

NPI

NOTES

AUTHORIZATION #

DIAGNOSIS
Essential hypertension
PAYMENT AMOUNT

JAMES L. SMITH
100 MEADOWLARK LANE
STEPHENSON OH 60089

No. 6789

Date Oct. 30, 2009

PAYABLE TO   Family Care Center

$17.60

Seventeen and 60/100 ———————————————————— dollars

Stephenson Bank
Stephenson, OH 60089

James L. Smith

021203347   0379 400 12   6789

PATIENT INFORMATION FORM

THIS SECTION REFERS TO PATIENT ONLY

Name: Uzwahl, Surendra	Sex: F	Marital Status: ☐S ☐M ☒D ☐W	Birth Date: 7/8/68

Address: 15 Main Street	SS#: 393-59-4392

City: Stephenson	State: OH	Zip: 60089	Employer: J.C. Penney (full-time)

Home Phone: 614-931-3715	Employer's Address:

Work Phone: 614-344-3118	City:	State:	Zip:

Spouse's Name:	Spouse's Employer:

Emergency Contact:	Relationship:	Phone #:

FILL IN IF PATIENT IS A MINOR

Parent/Guardian's Name:	Sex:	Marital Status: ☐S ☐M ☐D ☐W	Birth Date:

Phone:	SS#:

Address:	Employer:

City:	State:	Zip:	Employer's Address:

Student Status:	City:	State:	Zip:

INSURANCE INFORMATION

Primary Insurance Company: Blue Cross/Blue Shield	Secondary Insurance Company:

Subscriber's Name: (same)	Birth Date: 7/8/68	Subscriber's Name:	Birth Date:

Plan:	SS#: 393-59-4392	Plan:

Policy #: 393594392	Group #: 36	Policy #:	Group #:

Deductible $500	Price Code: A

OTHER INFORMATION

Reason for visit: Ankle hurt in fall	Allergy to Medication (list):

Name of referring physician:	If auto accident, list date and state in which it occurred:

Regardless of any insurance coverage I may or may not have, it is my responsibility to pay the entire bill. In the event that this office needs to obtain legal assistance in collection of any unpaid balance, I agree to pay costs and attorney fees, as allowable by law. I authorize the release of the above patient's medical records for billing purposes. I authorize payment of medical benefits to Dr. Katherine Yan, Dr. Jessica Rudner, or Dr. John Rudner.

Surendra Uzwahl	11/6/2009
(Patient's Signature/Parent or Guardian's Signature)	(Date)

11/6/09
DATE

Family Care Center
285 Stephenson Boulevard
Stephenson, OH 60089
614-555-0100

Dr. Katherine Yan
PROVIDER

Uzwahl, Surenda
PATIENT NAME

UZWSU000
CHART #

OFFICE VISITS - SYMPTOMATIC	
99201	OF--New Patient Minimal
99202	OF--New Patient Low
99203	OF--New Patient Detailed
99204	OF--New Patient Moderate
99205	OF--New Patient High
99211	OF--Established Patient Minimal
99212	OF--Established Patient Low
99213	OF--Established Patient Detailed
99214	OF--Established Patient Moderate
99215	OF--Established Patient High

PREVENTIVE VISITS	
NEW	
99381	Under 1 Year
99382	1 - 4 Years
99383	5 - 11 Years
99384	12 - 17 Years
99385	18 - 39 Years
99386	40 - 64 Years
99387	65 Years & Up
ESTABLISHED	
99391	Under 1 Year
99392	1 - 4 Years
99393	5 - 11 Years
99394	12 - 17 Years
99395	18 - 39 Years
99396	40 - 64 Years
99397	65 Years & Up

PROCEDURES	
12011	Repair of superficial wounds, face
29125	Short arm splint
45378	Colonoscopy--diagnostic
45380	Colonoscopy--biopsy
71010	Chest x-ray, frontal
71020	Chest x-ray, frontal and lateral
73070	Elbow x-ray, AP and lateral

73090	Forearm x-ray, AP and lateral
73100	Wrist x-ray, AP and lateral
73600	Ankle x-ray, AP and lateral
93000	Electrocardiogram--EEG
93015	Treadmill stress test

LABORATORY	
80061	Lipid panel
82270	Hemoccult--stool screening
82465	Cholesterol test
82947	Glucose--quantitative
82951	Glucose tolerance test
83718	HDL cholesterol test
85007	Manual WBC
85025	CBC w/diff.
85651	Erythrocyte sed rate--ESR
86585	Tine test
87040	Strep culture
87430	Strep screen
87086	Urine colony count
87088	Urine culture

INJECTIONS	
90471	Immunization administration
90657	Influenza injection, under 35 months
90658	Influenza injection, older than 3 years
90703	Tetanus immunization
90707	MMR immunization

REFERRING PHYSICIAN

NPI

NOTES

AUTHORIZATION #

DIAGNOSIS
Sprain or strain

PAYMENT AMOUNT

Family Care Center
285 Stephenson Boulevard
Stephenson, OH 60089
614-555-0100

11/6/09
DATE

Bell, Jonathan
PATIENT NAME

Dr. Katherine Yan
PROVIDER

BELJO000
CHART #

OFFICE VISITS - SYMPTOMATIC	
99201	OF--New Patient Minimal
99202	OF--New Patient Low
99203	OF--New Patient Detailed
99204	OF--New Patient Moderate
99205	OF--New Patient High
99211	OF--Established Patient Minimal
99212	OF--Established Patient Low
99213	OF--Established Patient Detailed
99214	OF--Established Patient Moderate
99215	OF--Established Patient High
PREVENTIVE VISITS	
NEW	
99381	Under 1 Year
99382	1 - 4 Years
99383	5 - 11 Years
99384	12 - 17 Years
99385	18 - 39 Years
99386	40 - 64 Years
99387	65 Years & Up
ESTABLISHED	
99391	Under 1 Year
99392	1 - 4 Years
99393	5 - 11 Years
99394	12 - 17 Years
99395	18 - 39 Years
99396	40 - 64 Years
99397	65 Years & Up
PROCEDURES	
12011	Repair of superficial wounds, face
29125	Short arm splint
45378	Colonoscopy--diagnostic
45380	Colonoscopy--biopsy
71010	Chest x-ray, frontal
71020	Chest x-ray, frontal and lateral
73070	Elbow x-ray, AP and lateral

73090	Forearm x-ray, AP and lateral
73100	Wrist x-ray, AP and lateral
73600	Ankle x-ray, AP and lateral
93000	Electrocardiogram--EEG
93015	Treadmill stress test
LABORATORY	
80061	Lipid panel
82270	Hemoccult--stool screening
82465	Cholesterol test
82947	Glucose--quantitative
82951	Glucose tolerance test
83718	HDL cholesterol test
85007	Manual WBC
85025	CBC w/diff.
85651	Erythrocyte sed rate--ESR
86585	Tine test
87040	Strep culture
87430	Strep screen
87086	Urine colony count
87088	Urine culture
INJECTIONS	
90471	Immunization administration
90657	Influenza injection, under 35 months
90658	Influenza injection, older than 3 years
90703	Tetanus immunization
90707	MMR immunization

REFERRING PHYSICIAN

NPI

NOTES

AUTHORIZATION #

DIAGNOSIS
Influenza

PAYMENT AMOUNT
$15 copayment, check #6130

BLUE CROSS BLUE SHIELD
340 Preston Boulevard
Columbus, OH 60220

PROVIDER REMITTANCE
THIS IS NOT A BILL
A PAYMENT SUMMARY AND AN EXPLANATION OF
CODES ARE AT THE END OF THIS STATEMENT

FAMILY CARE CENTER
285 STEPHENSON BLVD.
STEPHENSON, OH 60089

PAGE: 1 OF 2
DATE: 11/6/09
ID NUMBER: 36097869

PROVIDER: KATHERINE YAN, M.D.

PATIENT: BARMENSTEIN ELLEN

PROC CODE	FROM DATE	THRU DATE	TREAT -MENT	STATUS CODE	AMOUNT CHRGD	AMOUNT ALLWD	COPAY/ DEDUCT	AMOUNT APPRVD	PATIENT BALANCE
99211	11/4/09	11/4/09	1	A	30.00	30.00	.00	24.00	6.00
83718	11/4/09	11/4/09	1	A	35.00	35.00	.00	28.00	7.00
		TOTALS			65.00	65.00	.00	52.00	13.00

PATIENT: BLACK JO

PROC CODE	FROM DATE	THRU DATE	TREAT -MENT	STATUS CODE	AMOUNT CHRGD	AMOUNT ALLWD	COPAY/ DEDUCT	AMOUNT APPRVD	PATIENT BALANCE
99203	11/2/09	11/2/09	1	A	100.00	100.00	.00	80.00	20.00
		TOTALS			100.00	100.00	.00	80.00	20.00

PATIENT: FELDMAN STANLEY

PROC CODE	FROM DATE	THRU DATE	TREAT -MENT	STATUS CODE	AMOUNT CHRGD	AMOUNT ALLWD	COPAY/ DEDUCT	AMOUNT APPRVD	PATIENT BALANCE
99211	11/2/09	11/2/09	1	A	30.00	30.00	.00	24.00	6.00
80061	11/2/09	11/2/09	1	A	70.00	70.00	.00	56.00	14.00
		TOTALS			100.00	100.00	.00	80.00	20.00

PATIENT: JOHNSON MARION

PROC CODE	FROM DATE	THRU DATE	TREAT -MENT	STATUS CODE	AMOUNT CHRGD	AMOUNT ALLWD	COPAY/ DEDUCT	AMOUNT APPRVD	PATIENT BALANCE
99212	10/30/09	10/30/09	1	A	44.00	44.00	.00	35.20	8.80
71010	10/30/09	10/30/09	1	A	80.00	80.00	.00	64.00	16.00
		TOTALS			124.00	124.00	.00	99.20	24.80

STATUS CODES:
A - APPROVED   AJ - ADJUSTMENT   IP - IN PROCESS   R - REJECTED   V - VOID

BLUE CROSS BLUE SHIELD
340 Preston Boulevard
Columbus, OH 60220

PROVIDER REMITTANCE
THIS IS NOT A BILL
A PAYMENT SUMMARY AND AN EXPLANATION OF
CODES ARE AT THE END OF THIS STATEMENT

FAMILY CARE CENTER
285 STEPHENSON BLVD.
STEPHENSON, OH 60089

PAGE: 2 OF 2
DATE: 11/6/09
ID NUMBER: 36097869

PROVIDER: KATHERINE YAN, M.D.

PATIENT: LOMOS CEDERA

PROC CODE	FROM DATE	THRU DATE	TREAT-MENT	STATUS CODE	AMOUNT CHRGD	AMOUNT ALLWD	COPAY/ DEDUCT	AMOUNT APPRVD	PATIENT BALANCE
99211	11/2/09	11/2/09	1	A	30.00	30.00	.00	24.00	6.00
		TOTALS			30.00	30.00	.00	24.00	6.00

PATIENT: SMITH JAMES

PROC CODE	FROM DATE	THRU DATE	TREAT-MENT	STATUS CODE	AMOUNT CHRGD	AMOUNT ALLWD	COPAY/ DEDUCT	AMOUNT APPRVD	PATIENT BALANCE
99215	11/4/09	11/4/09	1	A	135.00	135.00	.00	108.00	27.00
93015	11/4/09	11/4/09	1	A	325.00	325.00	.00	260.00	65.00
		TOTALS			460.00	460.00	.00	368.00	92.00

PATIENT: SMITH SARABETH

PROC CODE	FROM DATE	THRU DATE	TREAT-MENT	STATUS CODE	AMOUNT CHRGD	AMOUNT ALLWD	COPAY/ DEDUCT	AMOUNT APPRVD	PATIENT BALANCE
99395	11/4/09	11/4/09	1	A	136.00	136.00	.00	108.80	27.20
		TOTALS			136.00	136.00	.00	108.80	27.20

PAYMENT SUMMARY		TOTAL ALL CLAIMS		EFT INFORMATION	
TOTAL AMOUNT PAID	812.00	AMOUNT CHARGES	1015.00	NUMBER	36097869
PRIOR CREDIT BALANCE	.00	AMOUNT ALLOWED	1015.00	DATE	11/6/09
CURRENT CREDIT DEFERRED	.00	DEDUCTIBLE	.00	AMOUNT	812.00
PRIOR CREDIT APPLIED	.00	COPAY	.00		
NEW CREDIT BALANCE	.00	OTHER REDUCTION	.00		
NET DISBURSED	812.00	AMOUNT APPROVED	812.00		

STATUS CODES:
A - APPROVED   AJ - ADJUSTMENT   IP - IN PROCESS   R - REJECTED   V - VOID

Index

Create Transactions button, 80
Customizing reports, 128–130
Cycle billing, 111

D

Data
  backup, 16, 48–51, 72, 95, 112, 130
  deleting, 40, 107, 148–149
  editing, 34–35, 40–42, 71, 102–103
  entering, 66–72, 78–95, 143–144
  saving, 26, 40, 80, 82
  searching for, in NDCMedisoft™, 43–46, 144–148
Data disk. *See* Student data disk
Data file, 16
Databases
  advantages of, 32–35
  defined, 16
  medical office, 16–17
  NDCMedisoft™, 16–17, 32–35, 43–46, 80
  searching, 43–46, 144–148
Date
  in appointment scheduling, 144–147
  looking for future, 144–147
  NDCMedisoft™ program, 29, 79, 144–147
  transaction, 79
  Windows system, 29, 116, 142
Day sheet, 116–119
  components of, 3
  computerized preparation, 35, 117–119
  defined, 2, 3, 116
  entering payments on, 8
  manual preparation, 16, 35
  printing, 117–119
  sample, 5–6
  sample report preview, 118
Default
  defined, 79
  transaction date, 79
Delete button, 40
Deleting in NDCMedisoft™, 40
  appointments, 148–149
  electronic media claims, 107
Deposit List dialog box, 91–94
  adjustments, 94–95
  Apply button, 92
  illustrated, 91
  using, 91–94
Diagnosis, defined, 3
Diagnosis codes
  on encounter form, 78
  ICD-9, 8, 17, 78
Diagnosis folder, 62–63
Dialog boxes, NDCMedisoft™, 23–28, 29, 40. *See also*
  Transaction Entry dialog box

E

EDI receiver, defined, 101
EDI Report, in Diagnosis folder, 63
Editing in NDCMedisoft™, 40–42
  claim information, 34–35, 102–103
  patient information, 71

Electronic claims. *See also* Claim management; Insurance
    claim form
  attachments to, 105
  audit/edit report, 106
  clearinghouse for, 101, 105–106
  creating claims, 101–102
  deleting claims, 107
  marking accepted claim, 106
  processing, 34–35, 101–107
  proofing, 105–106
  reviewing claims, 106
  submission procedure, 16–17, 104–106
Encounter form (superbill)
  charge transactions on, 76
  computerized preparation, 35
  defined, 3
  manual preparation, 16, 35
  procedure codes on, 8, 17, 80
  recording information on, 8
  reviewing completed, 76–78
  sample, 4, 77
  updating, 78
EPSDT, 65
Errors
  correcting, 34
  in creating claims, 107
  proofing claims for, 105–106
  reducing, 34
Established patient, defined, 56
Exiting NDCMedisoft™, 32, 48–51, 72, 95, 112, 130

G

General ledger, defined, 2
Go to Date dialog box, illustrated, 144
Guarantor
  defined, 3, 43
  patient/guarantor information requirements, 58–60

H

Head of household, 43
Health maintenance organization (HMO), 11
Healthcare ID field, 60
Help options, NDCMedisoft™, 30–32
Hints help feature, 30, 31
HIPAA Privacy Rule, 56
HIPAA Security Rule, 33

I

ICD-9 (*International Classification of Diseases,* Ninth
    Edition), 78
  described, 8
  in NDCMedisoft™ database, 17
Inpatient, defined, 79
Insurance Aging report, 122–123
  defined, 122
  sample, 123
Insurance carriers
  in case information, 63–65

in New Appointment Entry dialog box, 144
   searching for, 45–46
Program date, defined, 29
Providers
   defined, 2
   NDCMedisoft™ database information, 16

R

Receivables, defined, 116
Remainder statements, 109–110
Remittance advice (RA), 9, 91–94
Removable media device. *See also* Student data disk
   defined, 48
Reports in NDCMedisoft™, 116–130
   analysis reports, 119–121
   Billing/Payment Status report, 119–120
   collection reports, 123–125
   day sheets. *See* Day sheet
   designing custom, 128–130
   encounter form (superbill). *See* Encounter form (superbill)
   Insurance Aging report, 122–123
   list reports, 127–128
   Patient Aging report, 121–122, 123
   patient ledger, 5–8, 35, 125–127
   patient statement. *See* Patient statement
   Practice Analysis report, 119–121
   printing. *See* Printing in NDCMedisoft™
   superbill. *See* Encounter form (superbill)
Restoring data, 50–51

S

Save button, 40
Saving data, 26, 40, 80, 82
Scheduling. *See* Office Hours, NDCMedisoft™
Searching in NDCMedisoft™, 43–46
   for available appointments, 147–148
   for chart numbers, 45
   for other data, 44
   for patients, 44, 45
   for procedure codes, 45–46
   resetting, 45
Signature on File field, 60
Simulation, patient billing, 133–140
   office procedures manual for, 133–135
   source documents for, 153–263
   step-by-step instructions for, 135–140
Standard statements, 109–110
Starting NDCMedisoft™, 24–28
Statement management dialog box, 107–110
   creating patient statements, 107–110
   described, 107
   illustrated, 109

Student data disk
   backing up, 48, 72, 95
   copying, 23–24
   inserting, 23
   removing, 32
Superbill. *See* Encounter form (superbill)

T

Tab key, 45
Telephone numbers, entering, 67
Time of appointment
   in New Appointment Entry dialog box, 144
   searching for available, 147–148
Title bar, NDCMedisoft™, 17
Toolbar, NDCMedisoft™, 18
Transaction Entry dialog box
   Charge folder, 78–79
   Create Transactions button, 80
   illustrated, 41, 78–79
   MultiLink button, 80
   Payment Tab, 86–87
   Saved Transaction with Updates Information, 82
Transactions
   adjustment, 76, 94–95
   charge, 76, 78–85
   defined, 17
   NDCMedisoft™ database information, 17
   payment, 8, 76, 85–95
TRICARE
   described, 11
   Medicaid and TRICARE folder, 65
Type field, patient, 60
Type of Service (TOS) codes
   default, 79
   list of common, 46

V

Viewing in NDCMedisoft™
   backup data files, 50
   list reports, 128

W

Walkout receipts
   defined, 86–87
   printing, 86–87, 88
   sample, 87
Warning message, 24, 26
Windows system date, 29, 116, 142

Notes

Notes

Notes

Notes

Notes

Notes

Notes

Notes

Notes

Notes

Notes

Notes

Notes